Current Trends in
Lithium and
Rubidium Therapy

Current Trends in Lithium and Rubidium Therapy

EDITED BY

Professor Giovanni Umberto Corsini
Department of Clinical Pharmacology
University of Cagliari
Italy

Proceedings of an International Symposium on Lithium and Rubidium Therapy held in Venice, 29 September–1st October 1983

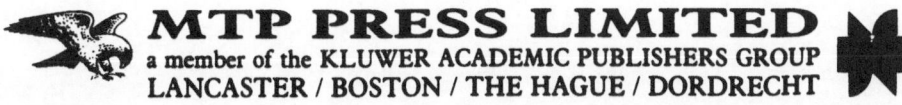

MTP PRESS LIMITED
a member of the KLUWER ACADEMIC PUBLISHERS GROUP
LANCASTER / BOSTON / THE HAGUE / DORDRECHT

Published in the UK and Europe by
MTP Press Limited
Falcon House
Lancaster, England

British Library Cataloguing in Publication Data

Current trends in lithium and rubidium therapy.
  1. Lithium–Therapeutic use
  2. Rubidium–Therapeutic use
  I. Corsini, G. U.
  616.89'18   RC483.5.L5

ISBN-13: 978-94-011-7320-9

Published in the USA by
MTP Press
A division of Kluwer Boston Inc
190 Old Derby Street
Hingham, MA 02043, USA

Library of Congress Cataloging in Publication Data
International Symposium on Lithium and Rubidium Therapy
  (1983: Venice, Italy)
  Current trends in lithium and rubidium therapy.

  Includes bibliographical references.
  1. Mental illness – Chemotherapy – Congresses.
2. Lithium – Therapeutic use – Congresses. 3. Rubidium –
Therapeutic use – Congresses. I. Corsini, Giovanni
Umberto. II. Title. (DNLM: 1. Lithium – therapeutic use –
congresses. 2. Mental Disorders – drug therapy – congresses.
3. Rubidium – therapeutic use – congresses.
QV77.9 158c 1983)
RC483.5.L5158 1983   616.89' 18   84-10042

ISBN-13: 978-94-011-7320-9   e-ISBN-13: 978-94-011-7318-6
DOI: 10.1007/978-94-011-7318-6

Contents

v

Preface

Lithium research and therapy needs to be continually re-evaluated on the basis of modern methodological approaches in order to shed new light on the mechanism of action and to improve therapeutic use.

This book, based on the proceedings of the "International Meeting on Lithium and Rubidium Therapy" held in Venice from September 30th to October 2nd 1983, is devoted to current trends in the pharmacology and clinical aspects of lithium and of a newly born therapeutic cation, rubidium.

The first part of this volume deals with modern trends in behavioural and biochemical approaches to the mechanism of action of lithium. A larger consideration is reserved for lithium therapy from a clinical point of view and includes re-assessment of long-term treatment with regard to serum levels, biological and psychological predictors, side-effects and new therapeutic uses.

A smaller section is concerned with some recent clinical studies on rubidium.

This volume should be an invaluable aid to all psychiatrists and those who work in the field of research of these pharmacological active metals.

G. U. Corsini

List of contributors

A. ALCIATI
Institute of Clinical Psychiatry
University of Milan
Milan
Italy

A. AMDISEN
Psychopharmacology Research Unit
Aarhus University,
Psychiatric Hospital,
Risskov, Denmark

P. H. ANDERSEN
Department of Pharmacology
University of Copenhagen,
Copenhagen, Denmark

F. ARENA
Psychiatric Clinic
University of Naples
Naples
Italy

J. BANNET
Jerusalem Mental Health Center
Jerusalem
Israel

L. BELLODI
Institute of Clinical Psychiatry
University of Milan
Milan
Italy

R. H. BELMAKER
Jerusalem Mental Health Center
Ezrath Nashim
Jerusalem
Israel

C. BENKELFAT
Mental Health Service
Hospital S.te Anne
Paris
France

P. BINET
Mental Health Service
Hospital S.te Anne
Paris
France

A. BOCCHETTA
Clinical Pharmacology
University of Cagliari
Cagliari
Italy

M. BOCCUNI
Institute of Internal Medicine
   and Clinical Pharmacology
University of Florence
Florence
Italy

G. BONO
Headache Centre
University of Pavia
Pavia
Italy

P. BONOMO
Department of Cardiology
University of Cagliari
Cagliari
Italy

C. BURRAI
Clinical Phamacology
University of Cagliari
Cagliari
Italy

H. M. CALIL
Department of Psychobiology
School of Medicine
Sao Paolo
Brazil

M. CASACCHIA
Institute of Psychiatry
University of L'Aquila
Aquila
Italy

G. B. CASSANO
Institute of Clinical Psychiatry
University of Pisa
Pisa
Italy

C. L. CAZZULLO
Institute of Clinical Psychiatry
University of Milan
Milan
Italy

R. CELLERINO
Clinical Oncology
University of Ancona
Ancona
Italy

S. CHAZAN-GOLOGORSKY
Department of Psychology
Hebrew University
Jerusalem
Israel

A. CHERCHI
Department of Cardiology
University of Cagliari
Cagliari
Italy

G. CONTE
Institute of Clinical Psychiatry
University of Milan
Milan
Italy

A. COPPEN
MRC Neuropsychiatry Research
   Laboratory
West Park Hospital
Epsom
Surrey
England

G. U. CORSINI
Clinical Pharmacology
University of Cagliari
Cagliari
Italy

F De LAZZER
Centre for the Diagnosis and
   Treatment of Tumours
Trieste
Italy

S. De LUYK
Scientific Institute Burlo Garofolo
Trieste
Italy

M. Del ZOMPO
Clinical Pharmacology
University of Cagliari
Cagliari
Italy

P. DENIKER
Mental Health Service
Hospital S.te Anne
Paris
France

M. FANCIULLACCI
Institute of Internal Medicine
  and Clinical Pharmacology
University of Florence
Florence
Italy

N. FERRANTELLI
II Laboratory for Clinical Reasearch
USL No.1
Trieste
Italy

R. FONZO
Department of Cardiology
University of Cagliari
Cagliari
Italy

P. FORNARO
Institute of Clinical Psychiatry
University of Pisa
Pisa
Italy

M.GASPERINI
Institute of Clinical Psychiatry
University of Milan
Milan
Italy

C. GAY
Mental Health Service
Hospital S.te Anne
Paris
France

A. GEISLER
Department of Pharmacology
University of Copenhagen
Copenhagen
Denmark

P. GOLAN
Department of Psychology
Hebrew University
Jerusalem
Israel

R. HAMBURGER-BAR
Jerusalem Mental Health Center
Jerusalem
Israel

F. N. JOHNSON
Department of Psychology
University of Lancaster
Lancaster
England

D. KEMALI
Psychiatric Clinic
University of Naples
Naples
Italy

R. KLYSNER
Department of Pharmacology
University of Copenhagen
Copenhagen
Denmark

S. KUGELMASS
Department of Psychology
Hebrew University
Jerusalem
Israel

M. LANFRANCHI
Headache Centre
University of Parma
Parma
Italy

A. LENZI
Institute of Clinical Psychiatry
University of Pisa
Pisa
Italy

L. LINDA
II Laboratory for Clinical Research
USL No1,
Trieste
Italy

H. LOO
Mental Health Service
Hospital S.te Anne
Paris
France

F. MACCIARDI
Institute of Clinical Psychiatry
University of Milan
Milan
Italy

M. MAJ
Psychiatric Clinic
University of Naples
Naples
Italy

G. C. MANZONI
Headache Centre
University of Parma
Parma
Italy

A MARELLI
Clinical Pharmacology
University of Cagliari
Cagliari
Italy

V. MAROLA
Institute of Psychiatry
University of L'Aquila
L'Aquila
Italy

G. MECO
Institute of Psychiatry
University of L'Aquila
Aquila
Italy

M. MELIS
Clinical Pharmacology
University of Cagliari
Cagliari
Italy

J. MENDLEWICZ
Department of Psychiatry
University of Brussels
Brussels
Belgium

E. T. MENICHETTI
Clinical Oncology
University of Ancona
Ancona
Italy

G. MICIELI
Headache Centre
University of Pavia
Pavia
Italy

S. MILANI
Centre for the Diagnosis and
    Treatment of Tumours
Trieste
Italy

G. MUSTACCHI
Centre for the Diagnosis and
    Treatment of Tumours
Trieste
Italy

G. NAPPI
Headache Centre
University of Pavia
Pavia
Italy

M. NEWMAN
Jerusalem Mental Health Center
Jerusalem
Israel

J. P. OLIÉ
Mental Health Service
Hospital S.te Anne
Paris
France

R. PALLA
II Clinic of Medicine
University of Pisa
Pisa
Italy

A. PENNATI
Institute of Clinical Psychiatry
University of Milan
Milan
Italy

C. PERRIS
Department of Psychiatry and
    WHO Collaborating Centre for
    Research and Training in
    Psychiatry
University of Umea
Umea
Sweden

M. P. PICCARDI
Clinical Pharmacology
University of Cagliari
Cagliari
Italy

C. PICCININI
II Laboratory for Clinical Research
USL No1
Trieste
Italy

U. PIETRINI
Institute of Internal Medicine and
   Clinical Pharmacology
University of Florence
Florence
Italy

R. PIROZZI
Psychiatric Clinic
University of Naples
Naples
Italy

M. R. PISANO
Department of Cardiology
University of Cagliari
Cagliari
Italy

G. F. PLACIDI
Institute of Clinical Psychiatry
University of Pisa
Pisa
Italy

A. PODDIGHE
Institute of Psychiatry
University of Cagliari
Cagliari
Italy

E. RAMPELLO
Institute of Clinical Psychiatry
University of Pisa
Pisa
Italy

M. REDA
Institute of Psychiatry
University of Cagliari
Cagliari
Italy

F. C. RODRIGUES
Federal University do Rio Grande
   do Norte
Natal
Brazil

E. RORAI
II Laboratory for Clinical Research
USL No1
Trieste
Italy

A. ROSSI
Institute of Psychiatry
University of L'Aquila
L'Aquila
Italy

N. RUDAS
Institute of Psychiatry
University of Cagliari
Cagliari
Italy

E. SACCHETTI
Institute of Clinical Psychiatry
University of Milan
Milan
Italy

P. SANDRI
Centre for the Diagnosis and
   Treatment of Tumours
Trieste
Italy

P. SARTESCHI
Institute of Clinical Psychiatry
University of Pisa
Pisa
Italy

F. SAVOLDI
Headache Centre
Univeristy of Pavia
Pavia
Italy

M. SCHOU
Psychopharmacology Research Unit
Aarhus University
Psychiatric Hospital
Risskov
Denmark

F. SICUTERI
Institute of Internal Medicine and
   Clinical Pharmacology
University of Florence
Florence
Italy

R. R. SILVA
Clinical Oncology
University of Ancona
Ancona
Italy

E. SMERALDI
Institute of Clinical Psychiatry
University of Milan
Milan
Italy

L. SMIGAN
Department of Psychiatry
Umea University
Umea
Sweden

M. TUONI
II Clinic of Medicine
University of Pisa
Pisa
Italy

A. VITA
Institute of Clinical Psychiatry
University of Milan
Milan
Italy

K. WOOD
MRC Neuropsychiatry Research
  Laboratory
West Park Hospital
Epsom, Surrey
England

Acknowledgements

This volume is based on presentations from a symposium entitled "International Meeting on Lithium and Rubidium Therapy", held in Venice, Italy in October 1983. We would like to thank the Istituto Farmacoterapico Italiano of Rome, who were the sponsors of this meeting, for their support. Further, we wish to thank Miss Anne Farmer whose assistance in the editing of this book was greatly appreciated.

Part I
Introduction and
Historical Review

1
Recent developments in lithium treatment and research

M. SCHOU

It is indeed an honor to be the first speaker of this symposium, and I would like to compliment our friends from Cagliari on having taken the initiative to, and carried the organizational burden of, what looks like a promising enterprise. Lithium has been dealt with at four symposia earlier this summer, on "Effects of Lithium and Antidepressant Treatment", on "Lithium Transport Research", on "Lithium Withdrawal Studies", and on "Trace Metals". The present symposium focuses on uses of lithium and rubidium in the treatment of illness, and I am particularly eager to learn the latest about rubidium as a therapeutic agent, a subject associated with many rumors but relatively few published studies.

The organizers have asked me to review some current interests and activities in our institute, but I am unable to report about therapeutic trials with rubidium, for we have given this drug only to primitive animals. In order to reduce the number of experimental variables *Christian Hoffmann* and *Donald Smith* (1,2) chose to study the behavior of jellyfish and planaria when exposed to lithium and rubidium. When lithium was added to the bathing fluid of the jellyfish in concentrations from 1 to 6 mmol/l, it led to an increased frequency of the rhythmic movement, while higher concentrations produced a decrease. Rubidium in all concentrations increased the contraction frequency. In the experiments with planaria, lithium and rubidium exerted similar effects; they slowed the gliding locomotion of the planaria as determined by the

number of lines crossed when the planaria moved on a graph paper with
1 X 1 mm squares.

There is obviously a long way from jellyfish and planaria to mentally ill humans, but *Hoffmann* and *Smith* suggest that studies on phyloge-
netically low animals might be of use in studying relationships between
neurophysiological and behavioral actions.

Our institute has given more attention to lithium as a psychotropic
agent, both to its wanted actions, therapeutic and prophylactic, and
to the unwanted effects (3,4), and we have been particularly concerned
with long-term treatment. *Amdi Amdisen* has reported about lithium effects on thyroid function as revealed by transversal and longitudinal
studies on large patient groups (5). These studies were carried out
with the main aim of examining the kidney function in patients given
lithium for many years, but since the studies have been reported on several occasions (6-10) and are in general agreement with the findings
of others, I shall not go into detail about them here.

The main outcome was that glomerular filtration is affected little
or not at all even when lithium is given for many years, but a number
of patients develop lowered renal concentrating ability leading to a
compensatory increase of vasopressin production and in some cases polyuria and polydipsia. The patients are accordingly at increased risk of
dehydration, and since dehydration may lead to a fall of the lithium
clearance and risk of lithium poisoning, the patients should be in-
structed to respond readily to feelings of thirst and to avoid fluid
depletion (11). We have also found it necessary to draw the attention
of surgeons and anesthesiologists to the occasional need for parenteral
administration of fluid to patients in lithium treatment, namely under
the following conditions: (a) When they vomit massively and hence lose
fluid without being able to supplement by drinking, (b) when they are
unable to drink because of long-lasting unconsciousness, and (c) when
they are forbidden oral fluid intake before surgery and narcosis
(12,13).

Tables 1 and 2 show what we suggest as minimum requirements for laboratory examination before and during lithium treatment (14). Many
hospitals will undoubtedly employ a more extensive test program, and
any abnormalities in the medical history of the patients or developing
during the treatment should lead to closer examination.

Table 1. Suggested minimum requirements for laboratory examinations
before lithium treatment

Urine analysis	Blood pressure
Serum creatinine	Electrocardiogram
Serum TSH	Body weight
Sedimentation rate	

Table 2. Suggested minimum requirements for laboratory examinations
during lithium treatment

Serum lithium every 2-4 months
Serum creatinine every 2-4 months
Serum TSH every 6 months

I would like now to draw attention to experimental work on rats
which has been in progress in our institute for a number of years and
which has led to important conclusions about the way lithium is hand-
led by the kidneys and hence concerning the mechanism of, and precau-
tions against, lithium poisoning.

Klaus Thomsen has shown that lithium is treated in a very special
way in the kidneys (15-17). The ion is filtered freely through the
glomerular membrane and thereupon reabsorbed in the proximal tubules,
including pars recta of Henle's loop, together with, and to the same
extent as, sodium and water, namely about 80% of the filtered load.
The remaining 20% are delivered to the distal parts of the nephron,
but here sodium and lithium are treated quite differently. While most
of the sodium is reabsorbed under hormonal control, very little, if
any, lithium is reabsorbed, and 20% of the filtered load are excreted
in the urine. In other words, the lithium clearance amounts to 20% of
the glomerular filtration rate. This means that lithium does not share
with sodium the rapid and finely regulated distal reabsorption, which
makes the excretion fraction of sodium, the sodium clearance divided
by the glomerular filtration rate, so variable. In contrast, the excretion fraction of lithium is very constant, about 0.2, both from
person to person and in the same person from time to time, and this
constancy of the lithium clearance is indeed a prerequisite for safe

administration of the drug. If the lithium clearance varied as much as the sodium clearance, we would be unable to maintain the lithium level in the organism within the required fairly narrow range.

However, the excretion fraction of lithium may fall under certain circumstances. Under conditions of manifest or threatening sodium deficiency or water depletion or both the proximal reabsorption of sodium is increased, and so is the proximal reabsorption of lithium. This leads to a fall of the lithium clearance, and unless the dosage is reduced or the administration stopped, lithium may accumulate in the organism and produce poisoning. It is this mechanism which is the common denominator for all those special risk situations during lithium treatment, which we have come to know from clinical experience: physical disease with fever, heavy sweating, low-salt diet, combined treatment with diuretics or non-steroid anti-inflammatory drugs, etc. A clear understanding of these renal mechanisms leads to more effective instruction of the patients and hopefully to fewer cases of unintended lithium poisoning.

It is interesting that these studies, which were motivated by interest in the mechanisms underlying the development of lithium poisoning, have provided a new and useful tool for kidney physiologists and nephrologists (18). Whereas previously proximal and distal reabsorption of sodium and water could be determined only through micropuncture studies in anesthetized animals, employment of the lithium clearance method, as proposed by *Klaus Thomsen*, achieves the same goal with a non-invasive procedure that can be used also in conscious animals and even in humans. The procedure consists in the administration of a small test dose of lithium, quantitative collection of urine, and serum lithium determinations at the start and at the end of the collection period. Hereafter the lithium clearance is calculated. Since all lithium that leaves the proximal tubules is excreted in the urine, the lithium clearance is a precise measure of the fractional proximal delivery of sodium and water. The reliability of the procedure has been substantiated by direct comparison with micropuncture determinations, and it is now being used increasingly in medicine and science.

In another series of experiments *Ole Vendelin Olesen* has drawn attention to the protection exerted by potassium ions against various nephrotoxic actions of lithium (19-23). When extra potassium is added

to the diet, rats tolerate long-term administration of lithium in doses that would otherwise lead to gastrointestinal disturbances, growth
retardation, and impaired renal ability to retain sodium and to secre-
te potassium and hydrogen ions. The additional potassium further prevents development of morphological kidney changes, lithium-induced
polyuria, and lithium poisoning. The studies illustrate how lithium in
several respects resembles, and in some respects differs from, diuretic
drugs, and they show that lithium interacts in a complex manner with
the renal handling of not only water and sodium but also potassium and
hydrogen ions. It remains to be seen whether these observations on rats
can be put to clinical use.

These glimpses of activities in our institute may be supplemented
by reference to work we are carrying out in collaboration with the Institute of Medical Biochemistry of Aarhus University. *Kristian Stengaard-Pedersen* and I felt that transmitter research, extensively pur-
sued with amine transmitters for many years, might advantageously be
supplemented by studies dealing with other transmitter systems, and we
have focused on cerebral opioid peptides and opioid receptors. Sensitive and precise analytical methods are now available in this field,
and hypotheses have been formulated concerning a possible role of these
transmitters in the pathophysiology of mental illness and the mode of
action of psychotropic drugs.

Until now we have studied the effects of desipramine and lithium on
opioid receptors in rat brain, and we have given the drugs in low doses
for a prolonged time in order to simulate to some extent the clinical
situation (24,25). The experiments seem to reveal that both desipramine
and lithium reduce the binding of ^{3}H-enkephalinamide, an opioid ligand
specific for opioid receptors and not destroyed by enzymatic action.
The two drugs differ as regards the parts of the central nervous system that are affected, but with both drugs the reduced binding of the
ligand appears to be caused by a lowering of the number of binding
sites, while affinity between ligand and receptor is unaffected. We
are not at present trying to interpret these findings in terms of animal behavior or drug actions on manic-depressive illness, but we hope
that the concurrent study of different treatment modalities, including
perhaps also electrically induced seizures, may provide evidence of
potential clinical relevance.

In conclusion, lithium is a valuable, if somewhat toxic, drug, with properties not fully shared by any other psychotropic agent. Studies on the mechanisms underlying its wanted actions and adverse effects may lead to safer and more effective use of lithium itself and perhaps to the development of new treatment modalities. Hopefully this symposium will bring increased insight and more efficient help for seriously ill patients.

REFERENCES

1. Hoffmann, C. and Smith, D.F. (1979). Lithium and rubidium: Effects on the rhythmic swimming movement of jellyfish (*Aurelia aurita*). *Experientia*, *35*, 1177-1178.

2. Hoffmann, C. and Smith, D.F. (1983). Lithium and rubidium: Effects on locomotion of planaria (*Dendrocoelum lacteum*). *Experientia*, *39*, 179-180.

3. Schou, M. (1979). Lithium research at the psychopharmacology research unit, Risskov, Denmark. In: Schou, M. and Strömgren, E. (eds). *Origin, Prevention and Treatment of Affective Disorders*. pp. 1-8. (London: Academic Press).

4. Schou, M. (1979). Publications on lithium from the psychopharmacology research unit, Risskov, during the period 1954 - August 1978. In: Schou, M. and Strömgren, E. (eds). *Origin, Prevention and Treatment of Affective Disorders*. pp. 9-26. (London: Academic Press).

5. Amdisen, A. and Andersen, C.J. (1982). Lithium treatment and thyroid function: A survey of 237 patients in long-term lithium treatment. *Pharmacopsychiatry*, *15*, 149-155.

6. Vestergaard, P., Amdisen, A., Hansen, H.E. and Schou, M. (1979). Lithium treatment and kidney function: A survey of 237 patients in long-term treatment. *Acta Psychiatr Scand*, *60*, 504-519.

7. Vestergaard, P., Amdisen, A. and Schou, M. (1980). Clinically significant side effects of lithium treatment: A survey of 237 patients in long-term treatment. *Acta Psychiatr Scand*, *62*, 193-200.

8. Schou, M. and Vestergaard, P. (1981). Lithium and the kidney scare. (Editorial). *Psychosomatics*, *22*, 92-94.

9. Vestergaard, P. and Amdisen, A. (1981). Lithium treatment and kidney function: A follow-up study of 237 patients in long-term treatment. *Acta Psychiatr Scand*, *63*, 333-345.

10. Vestergaard, P. (1983). Clinically important side effects of long-term lithium treatment: a review. *Acta Psychiatr Scand*, *67 (Suppl. 305)*, 1-36.

11. Schou, M. (1983). *Lithium Treatment of Manic-Depressive Illness: A Practical Guide*. 2. revised ed. (Basel, München, Paris, London, New York, Sydney: Karger).

12. Schou, M. (1981). Lithium treatment and preoperative fluid deprivation. *Br Med J*, *283*, 1253.

13. Schou, M. and Hippius, H. (1983). Lithium-Prophylaxe und operative Eingriffe. *Münch Med Wochenschr*, *125*, 705-706.

14. Vestergaard, P., Schou, M. and Thomsen, K. (1982). Monitoring of patients in prophylactic lithium treatment. An assessment based on recent kidney studies. *Br J Psychiatry*, *140*, 185-187.

15. Thomsen, K. (1978). Renal handling of lithium at non-toxic and toxic serum lithium levels: a review. *Dan Med Bull*, *25*, 106-115.

16. Thomsen, K. (1979). The renal excretion of lithium. In: Schou, M. and Strömgren, E. (eds). *Origin, Prevention and Treatment of Affective Disorders*. pp. 95-106. (London: Academic Press).

17. Thomsen, K., Holstein-Rathlou, N.-H., and Leyssac, P.P. (1981). Comparison of three measures of proximal tubular reabsorption: Lithium clearance, occlusion time, and micropuncture. *Am J Physiol*, *241*, F348-F355.

18. Thomsen, K. (1983). Lithium clearance: A new method for determining proximal and distal tubular reabsorption of sodium and water. *Nephron*, in press.

19. Olesen, O.V., Jensen, J. and Thomsen, K. (1975). Effect of potassium on lithium-induced growth retardation and polyuria in rats. *Acta Pharmacol Toxicol (Copenh)*, *36*, 161-171.

20. Olesen, O.V. and Thomsen, K. (1976). A preventive effect of potassium against fatal lithium intoxication in rats. *Neuropsychobiology*, *2*, 112-117.

21. Olesen, O.V. and Thomsen, K. (1979). Potassium prevention of lithium-induced water and sodium losing conditions in rats. *Toxicol Appl Pharmacol*, *51*, 497-502.

22. Olesen, O.V., Hestbech, J. and Thomsen, K. (1980). Potassium reduction of lithium-induced histological changes of the rat kidney. *Toxicol Appl Pharmacol*, *55*, 79-84.

23. Olesen, O.V. (1983). The effect of potassium on some nephrotoxic actions of lithium in rats. *Dan Med Bull*, in press.

24. Stengaard-Pedersen, K. and Schou, M. (1982). In vitro and in vivo inhibition by lithium of enkephalin binding to opiate receptors in rat brain. *Neuropharmacology*, *21*, 817-823.

25. Stengaard-Pedersen, K. and Schou, M. (1983). Opioid peptides and receptors in relation to affective illness: Effects of desipramine and lithium on opioid receptors in rat brain. *Paper read at symposium in Copenhagen, June 1983*, in press.

2
Lithium treatment of mania and depression over one hundred years

A. AMDISEN

John F.J. Cade, the Australian psychiatrist (1912-1980) (23) became
famous within the entire world of psychiatry when in 1949 he, apparently as the first one, published results which showed the lithium ion to
possess therapeutic properties against mania (8). His trial was open
and uncontrolled and comprised a limited number of severely ill, hospi-
talized, psychiatric patients. His results proved lithium to be thera-
peutically effective in all ten manic patients, while in six patients
with dementia praecox there was a recordable but unsatisfactory effect,
and in three chronically depressed, psychotic patients there was no effect at all.

Cade's results inspired the Australian researchers Noack and Trautner (36), Ashburner (4), Roberts (39), and Glesinger (17) to carry out
further investigations in this field. When Samuel Gershon (16) came into the picture and after his emigration to the United States came to
mark the initial development there, and when Erik Strömgren (41), who
was also inspired by the Australian pioneers, especially Noack and
Trautner (36), applied the idea of lithium's use as a psychotropic
drug in Europe, the pioneer time was in fact over for the contemporary
lithium era. But none of these authors had penetrated more thoroughly
into lithium's pre-history as Cade in his 1949-publication.

It was therefore Cade who got the credit for having been the one to
start lithium's era as a psychotropic drug.

In his famous 1949-paper he reveals that the English internist A.B.

11

Garrod (41) had seemingly been the one to introduce lithium salts in the 1850'es as a new contribution to the already at that time complex treatment of rheumatism; he also reveals that for a period up to 1900 lithium had been in widespread use against rheumatism, and he finds it furthermore noteworthy that several spas with a special reputation for treatment of nervous ailments were characterized by their lithium-containing mineral waters.

However, it escaped Cade's historical research that A. Ure (47) had introduced lithium carbonate into medicine already in 1843, i.e. 10-15 years before Garrod published his textbook in 1859 (11), and also that A. Trousseau in 1868 (46) as well as Garrod in 1876 (15) saw mania as one of the many possible manifestations of "brain gout".

Cade therefore did not realize that for as long time as 80-90 years before he published his results a presumably not seldom used treatment of mania existed, i.e. a therapeutic or, more often, prophylactic treatment of rheumatism, and that Garrod regarded a daily intake of 5-25 mmol of lithium salts as one of the most important, if not the very decisive, part of this treatment, even during completely symptom-free intervals (11-13,15). - The commonly used lithium treatment of to-day consists in daily doses varying individually from 8 to 80 mmol (1).

In recent history, the prophylactic use of lithium against depressions was first described by the English psychiatrist G.P. Hartigan, whose results were also based on an open and uncontrolled trial with a very limited number of patients (21,22). Also Hartigan was obviously ignorant of the fact that Garrod regarded "mental depression" as a possible manifestation of rheumatism, and it furthermore escaped his attention that the Danish neurologist C. Lange already around 1880 regarded "periodic depression" as a rheumatic phenomenon and consequently recommended a prophylactic treatment (27-31). Hartigan also did not recognize the facts that his famous countryman Alexander Haig (20) shared Garrod's opinion regarding the position of mental depression as a rheumatic phenomenon, that Haig (19) had included the more specific term "melancholia" in the concept of "gout" in 1888, and that he mentioned these viewpoints of his in all six editions of his famous textbook "Uric Acid" during the period 1892-1907.

The most likely explanation why the pioneers overlooked these historical facts is undoubtedly that during the decades after 1910 the meaning of the term rheumatism ("gout") had either undergone a change until almost beyond recognition or had become so much narrowed that in the years around 1950 neither of the terms "rheumatism" and "gout" would possibly suggest to anyone anything associated with psychiatry. It should be noticed that the Scandinavian pioneer M. Schou (42) must have been just at the point of discovering the truth of these historical facts when, referring to C. Lange's large review paper on the uric acid diathesis (30), he mentions that lithium had been in use against depression around 1897.

In the years around 1850 the main cause of rheumatism was thought to be an accumulation in the blood of "nitrogenized principles or calcareous salts" (48) and that this accumulation was caused by an inactive but first and foremost a luxurious living. The substances were deposited on the synovial membranes, in the urinary system, and in the arterial walls. The phenomenon manifested itself as individually varying diseases depending on which organ was most seriously affected. Deposits on synovial membranes led to often painful affections of the joints, in the urinary system they led to renal calculus and bladder stones, and in the arterial walls to a complex variety of organic disorders. When viewed over a longer period of time, the latter disorders were in the individual patient often combined with either urinary concrements, with joint affections, or with a family disposition to such affections. It was even thought that deposits in the arterial walls might result in senile gangrene (11,48).

Apart from the implication that such patients must take more exercise and restrict their luxurious living, it was thought that the excretion of these surplus substances was accelerated by local treatment and oral intake of various substances, especially salts, which stimulated the excretion through the skin, the gastrointestinal tract including the biliary passage, and through the kidneys. Looked upon in retrospective, it is noteworthy that one potassium salt, "silicate of potash" or "liquor of flints", was thought after oral intake to prevent the deposits, to redissolve them, and to promote their excretion (48). In analogy with Lipowitz' experiments (35) concerning the solubility of uric acid, Ure (47) examined the effect on bladder stones of, among other things, watery solutions of various salts. He found that a lithium carbonate solution was the most effective in reducing both

Table 1. Highlights of the first era of lithium in medicine

1841	*Lipowitz*: "Verwandschaft" between uric acid and lithium
1843	*Ure*: Treatment of bladder stones with lithium salts
1855	*Bunsen*: Production of pure lithium
1855-60	*Kirchhoff and Bunsen*: The first flame spectrophotoscope
1859	*Garrod*: "Gouty Diathesis" and acute and prophylactic lithium
1860-80	World-wide enthusiastic adoption of the "Diathesis" and its treatments
1876	*Garrod*: Mania and depression may be caused by uric acid
1886	*C. Lange*: Periodic depression, a new uric acid disease
1888	*Haig*: Melancholia may be caused by uric acid
1892-1907	*Haig*: Lithium alleviates gouty depression
1894	*F. Lange*: Treatment of severe depression with lithium carbonate alone
1930-40	Specialists are turning down the "Gouty Diathesis"
1930-83	*Survival of lithium drugs against rheumatism among non-specialists*

weight and structural density of a bladder stone. On the basis of these
results he postulated that the main role in the pathogenesis of rheumatism was played by uric acid. This viewpoint prospered when in the
1850'es Garrod repeated Lipowitz' and Ure's experiments, only this time
with removal of deposits on the articular surface of metacarpes from
dead patients who had suffered from rheumatism (11). Garrod then modified the hypothesis by claiming that not only inactivity and a luxurious living but also a disturbed uric acid metabolism in spite of a normal diet, or a reduced renal excretion of uric acid might be the cause
of rheumatism. In addition to urinary concrements and affections of the
joints he lists in his book from 1859 (11) as rheumatic diseases: epilepsy, periodic headache, periodic edemas, and anemia. He named his
hypothesis "Uric Acid Diathesis" or "Rheumatic Diathesis", and his
book aroused great interest. It was translated into German already in
1861 (12), republished in English in 1863 (13), translated into French
in 1867, and republished once more in English in 1876 (15). In the
latter edition he specified the concept of "Irregular Gout" as the designation of the vast variety of medical diseases which might be caused
by deposits of uric acid in different organs. The viewpoint was appa-

rently still the one that as good as any medical disease could be caused by an increased uric acid concentration in the blood or that it
could be a complication to a primary influence by uric acid on the organ in question. In the latter connection are mentioned diabetes mel-
litus and pulmonary tuberculosis as well as syphilis.

Table 2.   A few randomly selected examples of disorders, which might
have been caused by uric acid deposition according to Garrod
1876 (15)

Brain:	Mania, Depression, Hysteria, Hypochondri-asis, Headache, Epilepsy, Apoplexy
Spinal cord:	Pain and tenderness in the lumbar spine and pain in the legs
Muscular and nervous system:	Neuralgia, Cramps
Skin:	Prurigo, Pityriasis, Psoriasis, Eczema, Acne
Digestive organs:	Dyspepsia, Constipation, Diarrhea
Heart:	Palpitations, Irregular rhythm
Lungs:	Coughing, Asthma, Dry pleurisy
Kidneys:	Interstitial nephritis, Concrements
Eyes:	Conjunctivitis, Sclerotitis

The widespread acceptance of the uric acid diathesis as the basis
for the varied concept of "rheumatism" is illustrated by the fact that
during the last three decades of the century the hypothesis was readily adopted by outstanding scientists as, for example, Trousseau in
France (46), Cantani in Italy and Germany (9), Aulde in USA (5), Levison in Denmark (33,34), Pfeiffer in Germany (37), and Lange in Scandi-
navia (30) but first and foremost by Haig in England (20). As already
mentioned, "brain gout" might manifest itself as periodic headache and
epilepsy, but also as apoplexy and - of special interest in the present
context - as mania and "mental depression". In 1888, the explicit type
of depression "melancholia" was also included in the diathesis.

The Danish neurologist and pathologist C. Lange shared, as mentioned
previously, Garrod's viewpoints. In his private practice as a nerve
specialist he discovered what he himself considered a new type of depression of which he gave an exquisitely precise description at a meet-

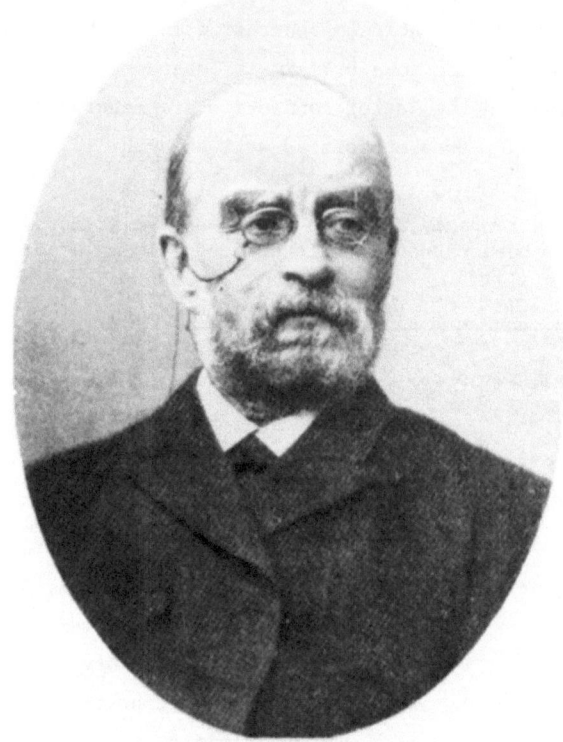

FIGURE 1   C. Lange

ing in the Danish Medical Association on January 19, 1886 (27-29,31).
- There can hardly be any doubt that what he then described were
slight endogenous depressions masked behind somatic symptoms such as
headache, dizziness, gastrointestinal symptoms, muscle or joint pains,
etc. - In Lange's opinion, this new disease was essentially different
from melancholia (38,43) and it was furthermore characterized by periodic occurrence, no progression, a relatively readily mobilized recognition and insight after unmasking, and a family disposition. It was
also always without psychotic features and was never sufficiently inva-
lidating to become recognized by psychiatrists in spite of its high
prevalence in the population. From several viewpoints, but especially
because of the clear periodicity, the inheritability, the frequent occurrence of urinary sediments, and the satisfactory effect of ordinary
rheumatic treatment, Lange classified his new disease with the large
group of rheumatic diseases. He fully agreed with Garrod that lithium

salts constituted a very important and perhaps the very decisive part
of the treatment; that this was indeed his opinion appears from the
fact that his brother, the psychiatrist Fritz Lange, in his textbook
"De vigtigste Sindssygdomsgrupper" ("The Most Important Groups of Mental Disorders") from 1894 (32) in the chapter on "Uric Acid Diathesis"
gives a representative example of disorders of this category: he reviews a patient with a moderately severe depression who responded twice, quickly and completely, to treatment with pure lithium carbonate
only.

The hypothesis was modified by Alexander Haig who claimed that the
sole pathogenetic factor was the high uric acid concentration in the
circulating blood. The primary reason for this viewpoint was that mi-
croscopy had failed to reveal the postulated deposits in the arterial
walls and organs (20). As regards lithium salts, he considered the use
of lithium carbonate a fault; acid salts should be used instead. He was
in some doubt as to lithium's efficacy, but maintained it among his
therapeutic measures as he found that lithium alleviated the depressive
effect of uric acid and produced a feeling of well-being; however, he
recommended the use of lithium citrate or lithium salicylate instead
of lithium carbonate, because these salts could remove the uric acid
from the blood, possibly through a temporary depositing in the tissues.

More reliable methods for examining the concentration of uric acid
in the blood had gradually been developed (18) and it had not been possible to confirm Garrod's claim of an increased concentration. The
Danish scientist Levison (33,34) therefore modified the hypothesis. He
thought that it was in fact a question of kidney affection caused by
urate deposits in the kidney tissue, and as neuronal reflexes emanated
from the kidneys to all parts of the body, this explained the variety
of rheumatic diseases.

Around World War I the uric acid diathesis was still commonly accepted as was lithium's connection with it (10), but technical developments and hence improved possibilities of diagnosing became fatal to
the reputation of the rheumatic diathesis among specialists. Urinary
concrements were excluded from the concept of rheumatism and arthritis
urica was isolated from it as an independent disease which was named
"gout" among laymen. In English-speaking countries the concepts were
altered semantically different: "gout" became synonymous with "arthri-

tis urica". In Danish, the term "rheumatism" in itself was hardly used any longer within medicine, and among laymen it was hereafter most often used to describe unspecific muscle, joint, and tendon pains.

However, once a concept has become widely and commonly accepted, it is hard to extinct even among experts in spite of a widespread understanding of its falsification (40,44). As late as in 1967, Tallbott wrote (45): "The designation 'gouty diathesis', so frequently used in the older writings of this malady, has not been abandoned even today". And in the 1981-edition of an English-Danish dictionary the term is still maintained.

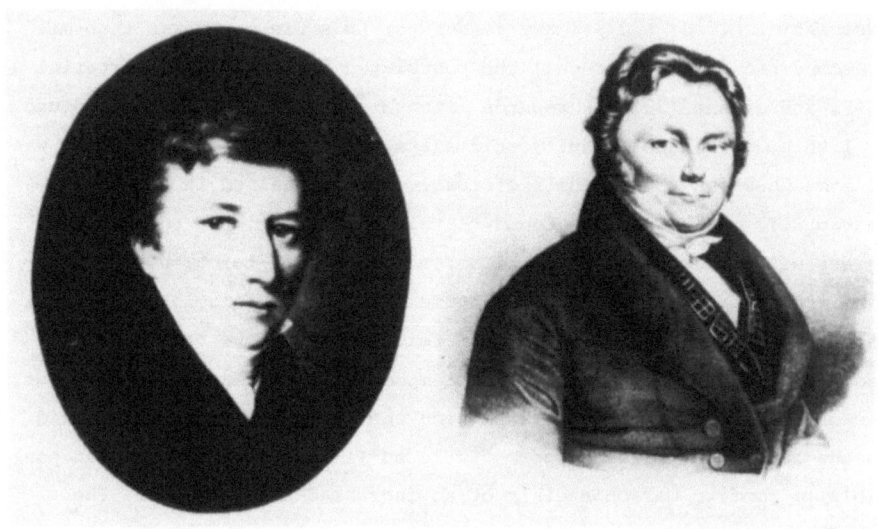

FIGURE 2   A. Arfwedson   FIGURE 3   J. Berzelius

Lithium was discovered around 1815 by the Swedish scientist August Arfwedson; he had been trained by Berzelius who coined the name of the new element (3,49). For the following several years no one knew of any physiologic significance or effect of it, although some people fastened upon the fact that lithium had been demonstrated in mineral waters from some spas with a special reputation for a favorable effect on kidney diseases (47).

Around 1840 the chemist Lipowitz investigated the properties of uric acid including its solubility. For instance, he compared the differences in the solubility power of potassium carbonate and lithium carbonate in identical weight/volume concentrations in water and found that the lithium solution was by far the most effective. He - and consequently later on Garrod - understood that this was the natural result of its higher content of carbonate caused by lithium's much less atomic weight, but he also found that boiling of uric acid together with a mineral containing about 4% of lithium led to development of lithium urate. He regarded this as a special phenomenon which, he thought, was due to a particular affinity ("Verwandschaft") between lithium and uric acid. The introduction of this, in reality false, concept of affinity significantly influenced lithium's further fate in the treatment of rheumatism, because Garrod (12) stressed this "Verwandschaft" as an important prerequisite for the use of lithium as an oral therapy. Ure (47) showed by in vitro experiments that a lithium carbonate solution was the most effective in reducing both weight and structural density of bladder stones, and he claimed that if such a solution was deposited in the bladder, it would be the most efficacious for treatment of bladder stones. But unfortunately the salt was very difficult to procure.

In 1855 R. Bunsen published a method for production of metallic lithium (16). At the same time the so-called Bunsen Burner with its low-intensity flame and very high temperature was constructed (7). With this instrument and with metallic lithium and pure salts of potassium, sodium, calcium, barium, and strontium as aids, G. Kirchhoff and R. Bunsen (25) constructed the first flame spectrophotoscope. With the high sensitivity of this instrument at hand they discovered new elements, for example rubidium, and they demonstrated that in practice lithium occurs ubiquituously, but for the most part as a trace element only (26). According to Garrod (15) the construction of this instrument was of decisive importance for lithium's fate as a medicinal drug, most reasonably because it had created possibilities for purity control during the production of lithium salts in their pure form and hence for a more rational production method. - A close connection between lithium in medicine and the flame spectrophotometer was re-established when in 1950 Talbott introduced the serum lithium concentration as a monitoring tool in guarding against lithium poisoning (44).

The easier access to both lithium carbonate and lithium citrate was the practical prerequisite for the success of Garrod's introduction of

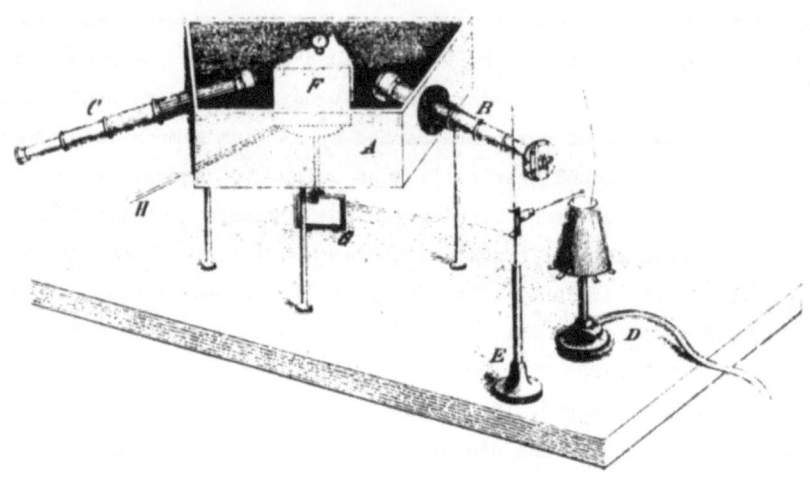

FIGURE 4   Kirchhoff and Bunsen's flame spectrophotoscope from 1860 (25)

oral intake of lithium salts as an important component in the treatment of rheumatism. As mentioned in the introduction, he recommended
lithium doses in the order of 5-25 mmol daily for the most commonly
used prophylactic treatment. In Garrod's opinion, however, lithium
salts were also worth using in short-term treatment of acute rheumatic
attacks.

As a further consequence of these conditions, some spas with lithium-containing water obtained a growing reputation for their putative
results in the treatment of rheumatism, and it also became a good busi-
ness selling lithium-containing artificial mineral waters (2).

Both lithium carbonate and lithium citrate had been included in the
first edition of the British Pharmacopoeia already in 1864. In 1873
Garrod drew attention to the fact that lithium carbonate could be used
as an antacidum, although he would not recommend its use as such. On
the other hand, he recommended lithium salts as effective diuretics,
a use which he considered very favorable in connection with the treatment of rheumatism (14).

It has not been possible to trace information about the magnitude of
the lithium consumption during the years when the popularity of the

rheumatic diathesis reached its peak, but it seems reasonable to suppo-
se that its variation was in rather close parallel to this popularity.
A very indirect reflection of the widespread use of lithium is found
in the varying numbers of lithium preparations available on the international market. The first edition of Martindale's "The Extra Pharmacopoeia" from 1883 includes 3 lithium preparations. Around World War I

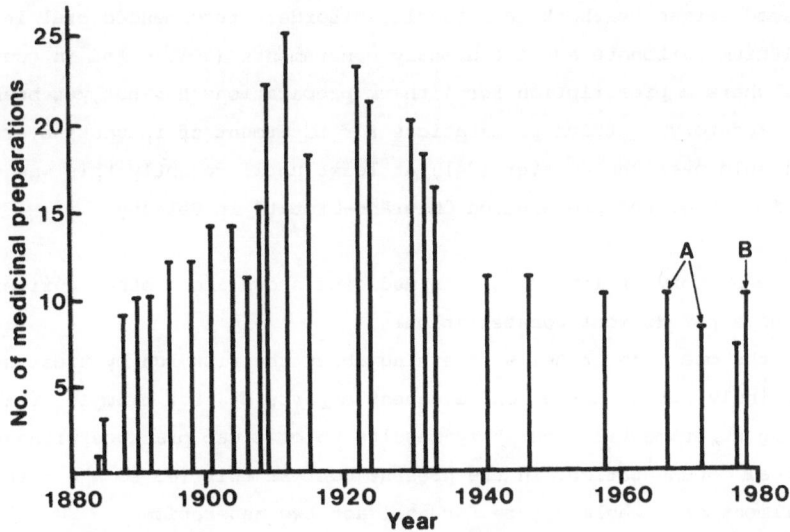

FIGURE 5   Number of lithium preparations available according to The
            Extra Pharmacopoeia ("Martindale").
            A: Lithium carbonate introduced against mania. Lithium citra-
               te against gout and rheumatism still maintained.
            B: Both lithium carbonate and lithium citrate against manic-
               depression.

the number has increased to about 25 different preparations, but in parallel to the still more declining belief in the clinical validity of
the rheumatic diathesis the number gradually decreases until around
1930 it reaches down to 15, and around 1970 only 8 preparations are included. In "Martindale"s 1967-edition lithium is introduced as a specific antimanic drug, but both in this edition and in the 1972-edition it
is still found worth mentioning the former use of lithium citrate
against rheumatism and as a diuretic drug.

The paradoxical survival of "the gouty diathesis" is thus reflected in the fact that medicinal lithium preparations have been available on the market during the last more than one hundred years, i.e. also to Cade towards the end of the 1940'es. Elderly Danish pharmacists have reported that the preparation against rheumatism "Urisalin" with a relatively high lithium content was sold over the counter in Denmark until 1965 when a prescription was made mandatory for all lithium preparations. It is also worth noticing that as late as in 1957 a highly esteemed German textbook on metabolic disorders recommended oral intake of lithium carbonate against urinary concrements (50). - And in countries where a prescription for lithium preparations has not yet been made mandatory, lithium preparations for treatment of rheumatism are still sold over the counter (24); at least until recently this was the case for, e.g. the preparation "Migräne-Orotat" in Germany.

The pre-history of lithium within medicine shows among other curiosities also a paradoxical constellation:

On the one hand it tells something about the risk run by trusting too blindly authoritarian and eloquent experts by, for example, transferring experimental laboratory results to clinical practice without clinical documentation. In the present context this led to a widespread·derailment of a whole sphere for at least two generations.

On the other hand, the adverse fate of C. Lange's preventive treatment of periodic depression (40) gives an example of the risk of losing a clinically valuable treatment modality by abandoning it without documentation, only because its original theoretical basis appeared to be false.

A more comprehensive and detailed survey of lithium's first era is given by F.N. Johnson in the first two chapters of his forthcoming book on the history of lithium treatment.

REFERENCES

1. Amdisen, A. (1977). Serum level monitoring and clinical pharmacokinetics of lithium. *Clin Pharmacokinet*, 2, 73-92.

2. Anonymous (1908). Lithia-Water. *The Chemist and Druggist*, October 31, 681-682.

3.   Arfwedson, A. (1818). Undersøkning af någre vid Utö Jernmalmsbrott förekommande Fossilier, och af ett deri funnet eget Eldfast Alkali. In: Afzelius, J., Almroth, N.W., Arfwedson, A., Berzelius, J. et al. (eds). *Afhandlingar i Fysik, Kemi och Mineralogi, Sjette Delen.* pp. 145-176. (Stockholm: H.A. Nordström).

4.   Ashburner, J.V. (1950). A case of chronic mania treated with lithium citrate and terminating fatally. *Med J Aust, 37(2)*, 386.

5.   Aulde, J. (1887). The use of lithium bromide in combination with solution of potassium citrate. *Med Bull (Philadelphia)*, 9, 35, 39, 69-72, 228-233.

6.   Bunsen, R. (1855). Darstellung des Lithiums. *Justus Liebig's Annalen der Chemie, 94*, 107-112.

7.   Bunsen, R. and Roscoe, H. (1857). Photochemische Untersuchungen. Zweite Abhandlung. Maasbestimmung der chemische Wirkungen des Lichts. In: Poggendorff, J.C. (ed). *Annalen der Physik und Chemie, Hundertster Band.* pp. 43-88. (Leipzig: Verlag von Johann Ambrosius Barth).

8.   Cade, J.F.J. (1949). Lithium salts in the treatment of psychotic excitement. *Med J Aust, 36*, 349-352 . (Republished (1982) *Aust NZ J Psychiatry, 16*, 129-133).

9.   Cantani, A. (1880). *Specielle Pathologie und Therapie der Stoffwechselkrankheiten.* (Berlin: Denicke's Verlag).

10. Galtier-Boissière, J. (ed) (1912). *Larousse Médical Illustré* (Paris: Librairie Larousse).

11. Garrod, A.B. (1859). *The Nature and Treatment of Gout and Rheumatic Gout.* (London: Walton and Maberly).

12. Garrod, A.B. (1861). *Der Natur und Behandlung der Gicht und der rheumatischen Gicht.* (Würzburg: Druck und Verlag von J.M. Richter).

13. Garrod, A.B. (1863). *The Nature and Treatment of Gout and Rheumatic Gout, 2nd ed.* (London: Walton and Maberly).

14. Garrod, A.B. (1873). Renal calculus, gravel, and gouty deposits and the value of lithium salts in their treatment. *Medical Times and Gazette, January 25, March 8, March 22.*

15. Garrod, A.B. (1876). *A Treatise on Gout and Rheumatic Gout (Rheumatoid Arthritis), 3rd ed.* (London: Longmans, Green, & Co.).

16. Gershon, S. and Trautner, E.M. (1956). The treatment of shock-dependency by pharmacological agents. *Med J Aust, 43*, 783-787.

17. Glesinger, B. (1954). Evaluation of lithium in treatment of psycho-

tic excitement. *Med J Aust*, *41*, 277-383.

18. Haicraft, J.B. (1885). A new method for the quantitative estimation of uric acid. *Br Med J*, *December 12*, 1100-1101.

19. Haig, A. (1888). Mental depression and the excretion of uric acid. *Practitioner*, *41*, 342-354.

20. Haig, A. (1892-1907). *Uric Acid as a Factor in the Causation of Disease. A Contribution to the Pathology of High Blood Pressure, Headache, Epilepsy, Mental Diseases, Paroxysmal Hæmoglobinuria and Anæmia, Bright's Disease, Diabetes, Gout, Rheumatism, and Other Disorders, 1st-6th ed.* (London: J. & A. Churchill).

21. Hartigan, G.P. (1959). Experiences of treatment with lithium salts. Paper read at Southeastern Branch of the Royal Medicopsychological Society (not published).

22. Hartigan, G.P. (1963). The use of lithium salts in affective disorders. *Br J Psychiatry*, *109*, 810-814.

23. Johnson, F.N. (1981). John F.J. Cade, 1912 to 1980: A reminiscence. *Pharmacopsychiatria*, *14*, 148-149.

24. Johnson, F.N. and Amdisen, A. (1983). The first era of lithium in medicine. A historical note. *Pharmacopsychiatria*, *16*, 61-63.

25. Kirchhoff, G. and Bunsen, R. (1860). Chemische Analyse durch Spectralbeobachtungen. In: Poggendorff, J.C. (ed). *Annalen der Physik und Chemie. Zwanzigster Band.* (Leipzig: Verlag von Johann Ambrosius Barth).

26. Kirchhoff, G. and Bunsen, R. (1861). Chemische Analyse durch Spectralbeobachtungen. In: Poggendorff, J.C. (ed). *Annalen der Physik und Chemie. Drei und zwanzigster Band.* (Leipzig: Verlag von Johann Ambrosius Barth).

27. Lange, C. (1886). Om periodiske Depressionstilstande og deres Patogenese. *Paper read at a meeting in the Danish Medical Association on January 19, 1886.* (Kjøbenhavn: Jacob Lunds Forlag).

28. Lange, C. (1895).Om periodiske Depressionstilstande og deres Patogenese. *Paper read at a meeting in the Danish Medical Association on January 19, 1886. 2nd ed. With an Epilogue.* (Kjøbenhavn: Jacob Lunds Forlag).

29. Lange, C. (1896). *Periodische Depressionszustände und ihre Pathogenesis auf dem Boden der harnsauren Diathese.* (Hamburg und Leipzig: Verlag von Leopold Voss).

30. Lange, C. (1897). Bidrag til Urinsyrediatesens Klinik. *Hospitals-*

tidende, 4. Række, Bd. V, 1-15, 21-38, 45-63, 69-83.

31. Lange, C. (1886). Om periodiske Depressionstilstande og deres Pato-
enese. *Paper read at a meeting in the Danish Medical Association on
January 19, 1886. - Reproduced in facsimile 1982.* Aarhus: Bogforlaget
DUO).

32. Lange, F. (1894). *De vigtigste Sindssygdomsgrupper i kort Omrids.*
(Kjøbenhavn: Gyldendalske Boghandels Forlag (F. Hegel & Søn)).

33. Levison, F. (1893). *Urinsyre-Diathesen. Gigt og Nyregrus.* (Kjøbenhavn: P.G. Philipsens Forlag).

34. Levison, F. (1896). Om Depressionstilstandes Forhold til Urinsyre.
Hospitalstidende, 4. Række, Bd. IV, 353-384.

35. Lipowitz, A. (1841). Versuche und Resultate über die Löslichkeit
der Harnsäure. *Justus Liebig's Annalen der Chemie. Annalen der Chemie
und Pharmakologie, 38*, 348-355.

36. Noack, C.H. and Trautner, E.M. (1951). The lithium treatment of
maniacal psychosis. *Med J Aust, 38*, 219-222.

37. Pfeiffer, E. (1897). Die Behandlung der Gicht. In: Penzoldt, F.
und Stintzing, R. (ed). *Handbuch der Therapie innerer Krankheiten.
Zweiter Band: Stoffwechsel-, Blut- und Lymphkrankheiten, Vergiftungen.*
pp. 22-56. (Jena: Verlag von Gustav Fischer).

38. Pontoppidan, K. and Lange, C. (1895). To psykiatriske Afhandlinger.
Anmældte af Dr. Knud Pontoppidan. - Et Par Ord om "den periodiske De-
pression" i Anledning af Prof. Pontoppidans Artikel "To psykiatriske
Afhandlinger". *Hospitalstidende, 49, 50*, 1204-1210, 1235-1238.

49. Roberts, E.L. (1950). A case of chronic mania treated with lithium
citrate and terminating fatally. *Med J Aust, 37(2)*, 261-262.

40. Schou, H.I. (1938). Lette og begyndende Sindssygdomme og deres Be-
handling i Hjemmet. *Ugeskr Læger, 100*, 215-220.

41. Schou, M., Juel-Nielsen, N., Strömgren, E. and Voldby, H. (1954).
The treatment of manic psychoses by the administration of lithium
salts. *J Neurol Neurosurg Psychiatry, 17*, 250-260.

42. Schou, M. (1957). Biology and pharmacology of the lithium ion.
Pharmacol Rev, 9, 17-58.

43. Steenberg, V. and Lange, C. (1886). I Anledning af Prof. Lange's
Skrift om periodiske Depressionstilstande. - Svar fra C. Lange. *Hospitalstidende, 3. Række, Bd. IV*, 629-648.

44. Talbott, J.H. (1950). Use of lithium salts as a substitute for so-

dium chloride. *Arch Int Med, 85,* 1-10.

45. Talbott, J.H. (1967). *Gout. 3rd ed.* (New York, London: Grune & Stratton).

46. Trousseau, A. (1868). *Clinique Médicale de L'Hôtel-Dieu de Paris. Tome Deuxiéme.* (Paris: J.-B. Bailliére et Fils).

47. Ure, A. (1843). Observations and researches upon a new solvent for stone in the bladder. *Pharmaceutical Journal, August,* 71-74.

48. Ure, A. (1844-45). Researches on gout. *The Medical Times, 11,* 145.

49. Vaquelin, M. (1817). Note sur une nouvelle espèce d'Alcali minéral. *Annales de chimie et de physique, 2(7),* 284-288.

50. Zöllner, N. (ed) (1957). *Thannhausers Lehrbuch des Stoffwechsels und der Stoffwechselkrankheiten.* (Stuttgart: Georg Thieme Verlag).

Part II
Mechanism of Action
of Lithium
and Rubidium

3
Some recent and some not-so-recent findings on the behavioural effects of lithium in animals

F. N JOHNSON

One of the most curious aspects of the history of lithium research
and therapy - certainly from the point of view of the psychopharmac-
ologist - concerns the role which animal behaviour studies have played
(or rather have *failed* to play) in the development of the practice and
rationale of therapy.   This situation contrasts markedly with that of
chlorpromazine, for example, or of the various clinically useful
benzodiazepines: these substances have been subjected to an intense
investigative programme by psychologists and others using a wide
variety of behavioural test situations and animal subjects, and the
findings have led to new conceptualzations of their modes of action.

This relative neglect of lithium has two aspects to it: in the
first place, little work has actually been done on the animal behaviour
effects of lithium salts; and secondly, such work as *has* been done
has either been totally ignored by psychiatrists and others, or has
been greeted as an interesting but largely irrelevant curiosity.

The dearth of experimental work is fairly easy to understand.
Lithium was introduced into therapy at a time when drug control
regulations in many countries were much less stringent than is now the
case, and so lithium salts were not subjected to the intensive testing
programme which is now mandatory before any new agent can be used
clinically.   The usual behavioural screening tests were not applied
to lithium for the very simple reason that the majority of such tests
had not yet been developed.   By the time that the test programmes had

become sophisticated and obligatory, lithium was already well
established as an agent of proven therapeutic efficacy and its
spectrum of side effects and contraindications was evident. The need
for laboratory-based testing was no longer there.

It has also to be remembered that the toxicity panic of the late
1940s and early 1950s led to the virtual removal of lithium from the
psychopharmacological scene just at a time when the behavioural
analysis of drug action was experiencing a boom due to the introduction of the phenothiazines and some of the newer anti-anxiety and
antidepressant agents (1).

The most important reason for the neglect of lithium, however, is
rather different. Recent work has shown that such behavioural actions
as lithium possesses are extremely subtle ones, and not such as would
readily show up in the majority of drug screening tests validated
against other psychoactive agents producing more powerful effects.
When lithium was subjected to such tests it tended to give negative
results, leading to the view that it was behaviourally inert. This,
coupled with the fact that when given to normal volunteer subjects it
had little or no effect on conscious experience, bolstered the notion
that lithium was a specific medication for affective disorders,
operating to correct, adjust or offset some presumed illness-specific
lesion. Since the lesion would not, by definition, be present in
either animals or volunteers, the absence of behavioural effects of
lithium outside the clinical context was both explicable and expected.
It was only when it was realized that a failure to detect behavioural
effects had more to do with the choice of the test situation than
with the specificity of lithium to manic depression that behavioural
testing began to yield results: this was in the early 1970s, twenty
years after the introduction of lithium into medical practice.

If the paucity of experimental data on lithium effects on animal
behaviour is easy to understand, the lack of impact which these
findings have had is less so. At the present time we are without a
satisfactory explanation of how lithium produces its clinically
useful effects: there is no single model couched in biochemical or
physiological terms which adequately accounts for the clinical
profile of the lithium salts (though individual models may go part of
the way towards this goal).

Why then, do psychiatrists so consistently ignore work which, up to
now, offers the *only* opportunity to develop a model which will provide
them with a rationale for the clinical use of lithium? For ignore it
they do: in articles written by psychiatrists in which the attempts
are made to derive a psychological model of lithium action no
reference is ever made to data from animal studies, *even though* such
data not only lend support to models based on findings from humans,
but provide much more precisely quantified information - and, what is
more, the animal studies predate the human studies often by as much as
a decade!

As early as 1972, for example, it was shown that lithium chloride
selectively reduced rearing activity in rats, and since rearing was
known to be responsive to environmental stimulation it was proposed
that the effect of lithium was to reduce the animals' responsiveness
to that stimulation (2). In further studies that same year it was
shown that when lithium treated rats were exposed on several occasions
to a novel environment and then had the lithium withdrawn, they
behaved as though they had never seen the environment before - unlike
saline treated controls which had habituated to the novelty (3).
This led to the suggestion that lithium not only prevented response
to stimulation but actually impaired the central analysis of sensory
information.

This is a hypothesis which has clear implications for a model of
manic depression, but if lithium does indeed reduce central information processing and is at the same time an anti-manic agent, then
one might hazard the suggestion that the manic state is characterised,
or even caused, by excessive central analysis of sensory output.
That idea was put forward in 1975 (4), but drew no reaction.

One reason for the caution with which data derived from animal
studies are treated lies in the problem of extrapolation of such data
from the animal to the human context. How, it is argued, can animal
behaviour be equated with that of humans? Moreover, the dose levels
and the dose regimes used in animal experiments often differ markedly
from those used in the clinical context. Clinically, lithium is
given chronically by mouth and in such a way as to keep serum levels
stable; experimentally it is frequently given intraperitoneally by
injection, in acute single doses which lead to transient serum lithium

peaks, and in doses which are usually higher than those which in
humans produce side effects or toxic reactions.

The answer to this kind of criticism is the simple one that what is
to be extrapolated from the animal work is not the data but the
hypothesis to which those data give rise, and hypotheses once formulated are independent of their origins, being refutable only in terms
of their predictions and not by reference back to the experiments
from which they were derived. Any experiment is a legitimate source
of hypotheses. To restrict one's work to a narrow range of subjects
(humans) and drug dose levels (those used in medical practice) would
be to throw away the opportunity of obtaining behavioural effects
which might lead to fruitful new ideas.

Psychiatrists are often too strongly wedded to the idea that
because a certain experiment was carried out on animals the hypotheses
to which the data give rise must necessarily be restricted to animals.
This is not so. A hypothesis is a hypothesis - neither human nor
animal but applicable, until refuted, to either.

It is, of course, wise to direct one's work with animals toward
test situations likely to give rise to useful and interpretable
information. There are several good examples of this in the recent
literature. Hoffmann and Smith (5) used the jellyfish *Aurelia aurita*
in a study of lithium effects upon rhythmic processes, finding that
lithium generally extended the period length of the rhythmic pulsing
of the jellyfish's bell. *Aurelia* was an ideal animal subject for such
a study: the hypothesis (that lithium may extend the period length of
rhythmic processes) is not however, confined to *Aurelia*: it is a
general statement abstracted from the specific circumstances of its
origin.

Engelmann (6) studied the effects of lithium on the periodicity of
petal movements in a plant, *Kalanchoë blossfeldiana,* and he and his
colleagues subsequently followed up this work with studies on a
variety of organisms including hamsters and cockroaches. When
Engelmann's work on *Kalanchoë* first appeared it was greeted with only
thinly disguised amusement by many psychiatrists. What possible
relevance could a water plant have to their manic-depressive patients?
The answer was simple: the water plant *qua* water plant had no relevance
whatsoever, but the *data* as the origins of a hypothesis about lithium

effects on rhythmic control processes most certainly *did* have relevance. Recent studies using human subjects have confirmed what Engelmann showed with his plant, namely that lithium has the ability to extend the period length of certain circadian rhythms, and these findings in their turn have led to a very powerful and influential model of manic-depression based on the idea of desynchronized circadian rhythms (7).

Smith (8) once argued that experiments on 100-day old male rats would only produce information capable of being extrapolated to 9-year old boys, awake at night, crawling on all fours and fed on a vegetarian diet. That is like saying that Engelmann's data on petal rhythms in *Kalanchoë* were relevant only to patients who had deteriorated to being vegetables and who lay all day soaking in a bath of lithium solution waving their arms about. It is not only to miss the point, it is to misunderstand the whole nature of scientific enquiry.

The hypothesis that lithium reduces the efficiency of central information processing, which was first advanced in 1972, has since received support from a variety of animal studies. Johnson (9) chose goldfish as experimental subjects in an experiment to study lithium effects on social behaviour, goldfish being eminently social animals and engaging in schooling behaviour. It was found that lithium treatment disrupted the social aggregation response of the fish. These results were related to an effect of lithium upon the analysis of social information, it being well known that the schooling response is mediated both by visual input and by sensory information arising from the fish's lateral line system of sense organs. In a subsequent study Johnson (10) established that responses to lateral line stimulation were indeed disrupted by lithium; it was found that even in the absence of visual cues goldfish would not enter far into a tapering channel (information about channel width presumably being encoded in lateral line responses to pressure wave reflections from the channel walls) but that after lithium treatment the fish would make much more adventurous entries. The hypothesis derived from this work was not simply that lithium impaired the processing of lateral line sense information (though this was *one* of the hypotheses, to be sure) but was the more general (and generalizable) one that the information processing effects of lithium are not sense modality specific.

Fish were again used by Johnson (11) to show that lithium had effects on behaviour only so long as the environmental stimuli controlling that behaviour were not salient (physically intense); in other words lithium was subtle in its action and the lithium effects could easily be overridden by environmental stimuli of suitable intensity.

The most recent findings (Johnson and Au, unpublished observations) show that in fish the behavioural effects of lithium on responsiveness to the environment are evident at dose levels of the order of one-tenth those needed to elicit clinical therapeutic effects in patients.

The net result of many animal experiments on lithium, some very recent and others not so recent, is the formulation of a very precise and detailed model of lithium action couched in psychological terms. What this model says is that lithium reduces the efficiency of central information processing of sensory input derived from all sensory modalities, provided that the stimuli giving rise to this input are low intensity, probably around threshold level. From this, a model of mania follows; this is that the manic state is one in which there is a *marginal* degree of central stimulus overprocessing. Johnson (12) has gone even further and has recently presented a very detailed model of the full manic-depressive condition, including both bipolar and unipolar forms and mixed depression-anxiety states. These hypotheses are derived from work *with* animals; they are not hypotheses *about* animals - they are relevant to people. Why, then, do the psychiatrists not take notice?

In recent years a number of psychiatrists have addressed themselves to the general question of the psychological mechanisms of lithium action and have carried out work on humans, both patients and normal volunteers, in an attempt to provide an answer. The conclusions reached, whilst tentative in the manner of their phrasing, are enlightening: lithium, it is suggested, may affect those aspects of human activity which are dependent upon the central processing of information (15). Where (and, more important, when) have we heard *that* before?

If we are serious in our claim to be investigators in the realm of *biological* psychiatry, we must accept that this means more than simply acknowledging the importance of biochemical and physiological data derived from humans; it means also recognizing that the human is an animal and, in an even broader perspective, is a living organism. Data from any living organism are potentially useful as a source of hypotheses which may then be applicable to the human condition. To ignore such information or to deny its relevance is to shut one's self off from a rich source of ideas. We should recognise too that a model of lithium action which is derived from data obtained by studying a variety of animal (and, if necessary, plant) species, is a model which is not linked to any one of these species: it transends the particular and becomes a general biological model. Such a model could well become a powerful tool in unifying the body of knowledge about lithium which has accumulated over the years but which so far has not been placed within a single conceptual framework. The key to a general biological model may lie in future experimental studies on animals: we might also find it lay in past ones if we were prepared to put aside our prejudices about the utility of animal experimentation in the search for an understanding of the ills of man.

References

1.   Johnson, F.N. (in press). *The History of Lithium Therapy*. (London: Macmillan).

2.   Johnson, F. N. and Wormington, S. (1972). Effects of lithium on rearing activity in rats. *Nature*, *235*, 159-160.

3.   Johnson, F. N. (1972). Dissociation of vertical and horizontal components of activity in rats treated with lithium chloride. *Experientia*, *28*, 533-535.

4.   Johnson, F. N. (1975). Depression: some proposals for future research. *Dis. Nerv. Syst.*, *36*, 228-232.

5.   Hoffmann, C. and Smith, D. F. (1979). Lithium and rubidium: effects on the rhythmic swimming movements of jellyfish (*Aurelia aurita*). *Experientia*, *35*, 1177-1178.

6.   Engelmann, W. (1972). Lithium slows down the *Kalanchoë* clock. *Zeitschr. für Naturforsch.*, *27*, 477.

7.   Wehr, T. A. and Goodwin, F. K. (1980). Desynchronization of circadian rhythms as a possible source of manic-depressive cycles. *Psychopharmacology Bulletin, 16*, 19-20.

8.   Smith, D. F. (1979). Six questions about lithium's effects on animal behaviour. In: Cooper, T. B., Gershon, S., Kline, N. S. and Schou, M. (eds). *Lithium: Controversies and Unresolved Issues*. pp. 936-944. (Amsterdam: Excerpta Medica).

9.   Johnson, F. N. (1979). Lithium effects on social aggregation in the goldfish *(Carassius auratus)*. *Med. Biol. 57*, 102-106.

10. Johnson, F. N. (1980). Effects of lithium chloride on lateral line responses in *Carassius auratus*. *Naturwissenschaften, 67*, 515-516.

11. Johnson, F. N. (1979). The effects of lithium chloride on response to salient and non-salient stimuli in *Carassius auratus*. *Int. J. Neurosci., 9*, 185-190.

12. Johnson, F. N. (1983). Stimulus processing and psychoactive drugs. I. The theoretical background and a model of affective disorders. *Int. J. Neurosci., 20*, 1-10.

4
Opposite effects of lithium and rubidium on neurohormone-stimulated cyclic AMP accumulation in rat brain

A. GEISLER, R. KLYSNER AND P. H. ANDERSEN

Lithium has been used for the past three decades for the treatment and prevention of recurrent mania and depression (1). The clinical specificity of lithium, which is well documented and generally accepted, implies a corollary biochemical derangement and makes it one of the first drugs whose action on the central nervous system may be studied in a logical manner.

In spite of numerous studies of the biochemical, neurophysiological, psychological, and clinical properties of lithium no unified theory of the therapeutic mode of action of lithium has been established and its pharmacological effects are still far from perfectly understood.

One strategy of research on the mechanism of action of lithium - and the etiology of manic-depressive psychosis - may be investigating and clarifying the influence of antimanic drugs versus that of antidepressants on central nerronal systems which may participate in the regulation of mood.

Such a strategy can include drugs which can precipitate depression, e.g. reserpine, or elation, e.g. amphetamine, or drugs which have antimanic properties, e.g. lithium in comparison with drugs used against depression.

Historically, the "monoamine hypothesis of affective disorders" was proposed on the basis of the pharmacological effects of reserpine and antidepressant drugs in relation to
their clinical effects (2).

Among the various hypotheses concerning the mode of action
of lithium, the aim of one line of research is to elucidate
the theory that lithium exerts its therapeutic actions by
an interference with the regulation of the density of cerebral noradrenergic receptors and/or their function, e.g. the
activity of the noradrenaline-sensitive adenylate cyclase in
nervous tissue.

As described below, several studies have shown that lithium
in vitro and in vivo, i.e. during chronic treatment and
within the therapeutic range, can inhibit adrenergic stimulation of cyclic AMP formation (3). Other studies suggest
that lithium may act on the processes regulating receptor
adaptability in this system (4).

In addition, several groups have demonstrated that various
antidepressant treatments such as polycyclic antidepressants, monoamine oxidase inhibitors and electroconvulsive
therapy reduce the density and the function of central beta-
adrenergic receptors measured by binding studies and cyclic
AMP formation (5). In contrast, the depression-provoking
drug reserpine has an opposite effect, i.e. chronic treatment with reserpine increases the number of brain beta-
adrenergic receptors and the adrenergic-stimulated cyclic
AMP synthesis (6).

A relationship between mood-modifying drugs and alterations
in cerebral adrenergic receptor binding and responsiveness
of the associated adenylate cyclase might be an important
research area which may contribute to our understanding of
the drugs used against affective illness.

Given the possibility that lithium may exert its antimanic
effects by inhibiting the cerebral noradrenaline-stimulated
adenylate cyclase activity, it was assumed that one test of

this theory would be an opposite response, i.e. a stimulation of adenylate cyclase by rubidium which seems to possess antidepressant properties (7) and an ability to prolong the period of mania (8). Furthermore, such a study could contribute to our understanding of the very complex regulation of the activity of adenylate cyclase.

According to the above-mentioned observations and notions the present communication will be divided into four sections:

1. The general structure, regulation and function of adenylate cyclase.
2. The influence of lithium in vitro and in vivo on adenylate cyclase activity.
3. Effects of rubidium in vitro on cerebral adrenoceptor-associated adenylate cyclase activity.
4. Discussion.

1. The general structure, regulation and function of adenylate cyclase.

At least three separate membrane-bound entities constitute hormone- and neurotransmitter-sensitive adenylate cyclases which are information transfer systems conveying extracellular stimuli (first messenger) into cyclic AMP, an intracellular signal or second messenger.

As shown in figure 1, the enzyme system consists of the receptor (R) located at the outside of the cell membrane, the catalytic subunit of the enzyme (AC) bearing the site that converts ATP to cyclic AMP, and a guanine nucleotide-binding regulatory component (G/Fs) that transfers the hormonal stimulus from the receptor to the catalytic subunit, thereby increasing the cyclic AMP synthesis. The generated cyclic AMP regulates the activity of intracellular protein kinases.

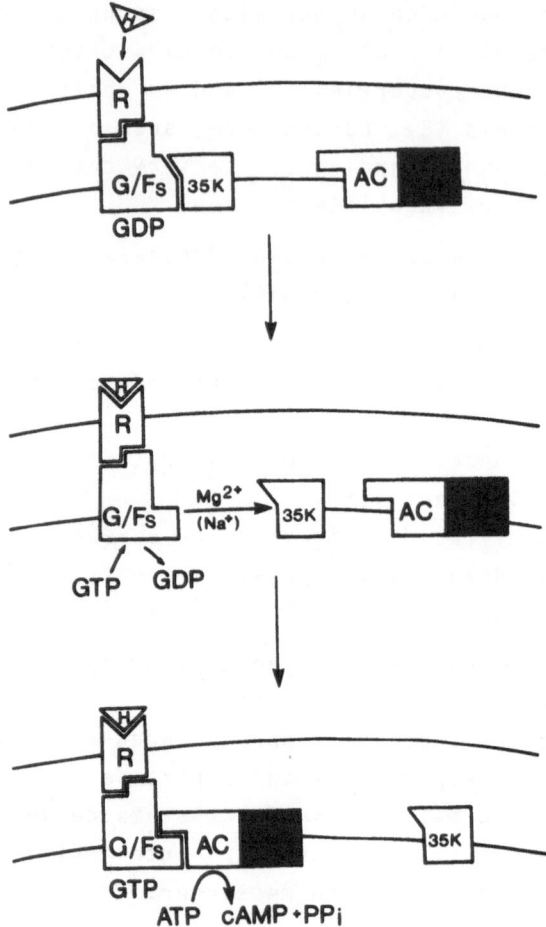

FIGURE 1   A schematic diagram of the interaction of the components in
the adenylate cyclase system. See text for further explanation

The cerebral adenylate cyclase is sensitive, depending on the
species and the brain region studied, to various neurotransmitters, e.g. noradrenaline, dopamine, serotonin, and histamine. Putative neurotransmitters or neuromodulators such as
adenosine, enkephalins, vasopressin, and vasoactive intesti-
nal polypeptide may also activate or interfere with the regulation of brain adenylate cyclase (9).

The separate components of the enzyme system are mobile within the cell membrane. When an agonist, e.g. noradrenaline, binds to the specific receptor, an interaction between the receptor protein and the G/Fs protein occurs. This complex, involving an association of hormone (H), receptor and the G/Fs protein which serves as an intermediate through which hormones stimulate the rate of activation of adenylate cyclase, is also affected by guanine nucleotides. Antagonists do not induce the functional association of the receptor and the G/Fs protein and, therefore, do not stimulate the catalytic subunit. Recent studies have shown that the G/Fs is a heterodimer which contains a subunit ranging in size from 45 K to 55 K daltons; this subunit seems to be the component through which hormones and neurotransmitters, guanine nucleotides and fluoride exert their activation of adenylate cyclase. The other subunit is a 35 K dalton component which seems to act as an inhibitor of the 45 K (55 K) subunit.

A variety of evidence has shown that magnesium in millimolar concentrations and calcium in the micromolar range can stimulate the adenylate cyclase activity by interacting with various allosteric binding sites. The component through which the divalent ions stimulate adenylate cyclase is not conclusively demonstrated. On the basis of suggestive evidence Rodbell has put forward the hypothesis that the 35 K subunit may contain sites for divalent cations (10). However, the question remains open whether sites for divalent cations are also associated with the catalytic moiety (indicated in Figure 1 by the black area on AC).

Shown schematically and simplified in Figure 1 is the integrative events of hormonal stimulation of adenylate cyclase. Further, it can be seen that magnesium (and possibly also sodium) among other effects appears to play a role for the dissociation of the two subunits of the "coupling" protein G/Fs and consequently participates in the regulation of hormonal stimulation of the enzyme.

A large body of evidence supports that various other substances, e.g. calmodulin, phospholipids, prostaglandins,
purines, neuropeptides, and possibly other unknown substances participate in the regulation or modulation of this
composite system which transfers information from the receptor to the metabolic system of the cell through cyclic
AMP and cyclic AMP-dependent protein kinases. Consequently,
interpretation of data concerning drug influences on the
adenylate cyclase system is impeded by the mentioned variety
of regulatory components and agents.

2. Influence of lithium in vitro and in vivo on cerebral
   adenylate cyclase.
In the introduction some considerations concerning the action of lithium on adenylate cyclase was briefly mentioned.
This section will review selected studies on the inhibitory
effect on adenylate cyclase activity by lithium. Several
studies using neuronal (11) as well as non-neuronal tissues
(12) have shown that high and toxic concentrations of lithium are necessary to produce a significant reduction in
hormone-stimulated enzyme activity in membraneous preparations. In brain homogenates the dopamine-sensitive adenylate cyclase from striatum can be consistenly and repro-
ducibly activated by the appropriate neurohormone. As seen
in Table I, 10 mM of lithium chloride was a prerequisite
of achieving an inhibitory effect of the enzyme.

Table I. Effect of increasing concentrations of lithium on adenylate cyclase activity in homogenized rat striatum.

Addition mM		Increase due to
LiCl	NaCl	dopamine 10^{-4} M
0	20	20.8 ± 4.1
1	19	19.5 ± 0.7
2	18	18.8 ± 1.1
5	15	17.6 ± 1.6
10	10	12.5 ± 1.3^{o}
20	0	12.7 ± 1.2^{o}

Results are expressed as pmoles cAMP formed/2 mg tissue/2.5 min. The unstimulated activity in the presence of 20 mM NaCl was $34.6 \pm$ pmoles cAMP formed/2 mg tissue/2.5.

$^{o}p < 0.05$ compared with 20 mM NaCl.

Mean $\pm$ S.E.M. n = 7. Data from Geisler and Klysner (13).

However, this insensitivity of the adenylate cyclase in homogenates to lithium-induced inhibition is not seen in preparations containing intact cells. Thus, by using intact tissue preparations, i.e. brain slices (14) or "liquified slices" (15), lithium in concentrations of 1-2 mM has been found to inhibit significantly neurohormone-stimulated cyclic AMP accumulation in vitro. These experiments have been performed in rabbit and rat cortex (16), rabbit retina (17), and rat limbic forebrain (18). Furthermore, such studies have provided consistent evidence that lithium does not exert effects on the unstimulated adenylate cyclase activity. Only very few studies, e.g. Gagnon (19), have shown that lithium in vitro can inhibit unstimulated cyclic AMP accumulation in intact cell preparations. Such discrepancies could, in fact, be due to differences in experimental conditions causing a variation in effects of endogenous activators which may contribute to the so-called "unstimulated activity".

Due to the narrow therapeutic range of lithium (0.6-1.2 mM) and the time-response relation of the therapeutic effects of lithium treatment it is of great importance that chronic lithium treatment, giving plasma concentrations within the accepted therapeutic range, has been shown to inhibit neuro-hormone-stimulated cyclic AMP accumulation. Belmaker and co-workers (20) have observed that in lithium-treated rats, having a mean plasma lithium concentration of 1.73 mM, the noradrenaline-induced cyclic AMP accumulation was reduced by more than 70%. In the same study no supersensitivity, measured by increased accumulation of cyclic AMP in response to noradrenaline, was demonstrable after cessation of long-term lithium treatment. In a subsequent study the same group observed that lithium treatment giving a plasma lithium level of 0.4 mM can prevent the reserpine-induced rise in noradrenaline-induced cyclic AMP accumulation, whereas no directly inhibitory effect of this low lithium concentration on the activity of the enzyme was found (21).

The inhibitory effect of lithium on cyclic AMP formation has also been demonstrated in man undergoing chronic lithium treatment. Thus, the PGE_1-induced cyclic AMP accumulation in platelets was reduced in patients having lithium levels in the plasma within the therapeutic range (22). Interestingly, the same study also showed that the noradrenaline-produced inhibition on the PGE_1-stimulated cyclic AMP accumulation was reduced during lithium therapy, suggesting a site of action of lithium common to stimulation and inhibition of the enzyme.

In man, rises of plasma cyclic AMP produced by infusion of isoprenaline (23) and adrenaline injections (24) were reduced by lithium treatment.

These - and other studies - have shown that lithium inhibits
the stimulation of cerebral beta-adrenoceptor associated adenylate cyclase. Observed interactions of lithium with other
hormone-stimulated adenylate cyclases from peripheral organs,
e.g. the thyroid and the renal medulla which produce typical
and specific side effects of lithium, support the hypothesis
that chronic and conventional lithium administration might
interfere with some, but presumably not all, adenylate cyclases. Thus, lithium does not inhibit glucagon-stimulated
cyclic AMP formation (25).

The fact that lithium during chronic treatment inhibits noradrenaline-stimulated cyclic AMP accumulation in brain tissue
does not, of course, imply that this effect is related to
its mode of action. The precise location and function, including their role for mood regulation, of the involved
beta-adrenoceptors remain to be determined. Some indirect
support of the assumption that changes in beta-adrenoceptors
are disturbed during manic-depressive fluctuations are the
multitude of studies showing down-regulation of cerebral
beta-adrenoceptors by various antidepressant treatment modalities (26).

The many observations showing that lithium inhibits hormonal activity of some adenylate cyclases may compose a set
of information which increase our possibilities for a better
understanding of the mechanism by which lithium interferes
with enzyme. Further, as the effect of lithium is selective,
i.e. only inhibiting the hormonal stimulation of the enzyme,
these investigations may be useful in our attempts to elucidate the regulatory processes involved in the function
of adenylate cyclase.

Some common and consistent effects of lithium on the activity of adenylate cyclase systems are:

1. Basal or unstimulated enzyme activities are usually unaffected, even by very high lithium concentrations in
   vitro and in vivo.

2. The fluoride stimulation (which can only be demonstrated in membraneous preparations) is only suppressed by lithium in high and toxic concentrations.

3. The inhibition by lithium has been shown, in disrupted cells and intact cell preparations, to be mainly of the non-competitive type.

4. Adenylate cyclase situated within the undisturbed membrane and therefore measured as cyclic AMP accumulation seems to be more sensitive to lithium than the enzymatic activity determined in membrane preparations.

5. Lithium _in vivo_ may have a dual action on the receptor-adenylate cyclase system. In concentrations about and above 1 mM in the plasma lithium can prevent drugs - and lesion-induced increases in receptor density (for review see 27), whereas lower plasma lithium concentrations (0.4-0.6 mM) only impair the enhanced transfer of the hormone-receptor stimulus to the catalytic subunit.

6. The inhibitory effect of lithium on cyclic AMP formation is, also during _in vitro_ conditions, time-dependent. This time-dependence varies from tissue, possibly due to differences in lithium transport. Thus, in intact rat brain preparations such as slices and synaptosomes the maximal inhibition is achieved in about 10 minutes. In isolated human platelets about 2 hours preincubation in a lithium-containing buffer is necessary to obtain the maximal inhibitory effect on cyclic AMP accumulation.

7. The inhibitory effect of lithium on adenylate cyclase activity is antagonized dose-dependently by magnesium and, as described in the next section, by rubidium.

8. A few recent studies suggest that human brain tissue may be more sensitive to lithium than cerebral tissue from experimental animals, e.g. the rat.

9. Chronic lithium treatment increases high affinity phos-
   phodiesterase activity in rat cerebral cortex and limbic
   forebrain.

The above-mentioned "profile" of the influence of lithium on
adenylate cyclase activity may allow the following assump-
tions concerning the mechanism by which lithium reduces hormonal activation of adenylate cyclase.

The site of action of lithium seems to be located intracel-
lularly, presumably within the plasma membrane. A direct
effect of lithium on the receptor protein seems unlikely,
since lithium alone has no effect on the number and binding
affinity of the adrenoceptors. Similarly, there is no evidence supporting an influence on the catalytic subunit as
basal enzyme activities are unaffected by lithium in vitro
and in vivo.

The non-competitive type of inhibition, the greater sensitivity to lithium of adenylate cyclases situated within an
intact membrane and the selectivity, i.e. only hormonal stimulation is suppressed, support that the site of action is
located "between" the receptor and the catalytic moiety,
thereby interfering with the transfer of the hormone stimulus through the membrane.

In the discussion our speculations concerning the effects
of lithium are further elaborated.

3. Effects of rubidium in vitro on cerebral adrenoceptor-
   associated adenylate cyclase activity.
Rubidium belongs, as lithium, to group IA of the periodic
system, but is one of the heavier alkali metals. Therefore,
in view of the therapeutic efficacy of lithium against mood
disorders, it would seem natural to investigate the effect
of rubidium on behaviour and brain biochemistry as well.

A growing number of experiments on animals have shown that rubidium has a unique neuropharmacological profile of effects which are opposite to the effects of lithium. Thus, it has been shown that rubidium, in contrast to lithium, given to rats for 10 days facilitates the turnover of noradrenaline (28). Further, it has been shown that rubidium enhances the presynaptic release of noradrenaline (29), whereas lithium has been demonstrated to increase the uptake of noradrenaline into synaptosomes.

Besides rubidium and lithium seem to have opposite effects on the EEG and behaviour. Thus, Meltzer et al. (30) have reported that rubidium increased the prevalent frequency of EEG in monkeys which also showed hyperactivity and aggressiveness. In contrast, lithium has been shown to slow the EEG and reduce hyperactivity (31).

Carroll & Sharp observed that morphine activity in mice was antagonized by pretreatment with lithium but potentiated by treatment with rubidium (32).

Because the changes produced by rubidium on noradrenaline turnover, EEG and behaviour can be described as "opposite" to those produced by lithium, it has been hypothesized that rubidium may have an application in the treatment of depression (33). Interestingly, Jenner has observed that rubidium can prolong or exaggerate manic states (34).

Due to the neurochemical, behavioural, and clinical properties of rubidium we decided to investigate its effect on the cerebral adenylate cyclase in comparison with lithium. Until now, we have only performed in vitro investigations using rat brain cortical slices. The methods used have been described in detail elsewhere (35). However, it should be noted that the cortical slices were preincubated for 40 minutes with cations as indicated before the incubation period.

As seen in Figure 2, lithium in a concentration of 2 mM reduced significantly ($p < 0.05$) stimulation of the enzyme
with increasing concentrations of noradrenaline. The inhibition by lithium was of the non-competitive type suggesting
a site of action beyond the receptor.

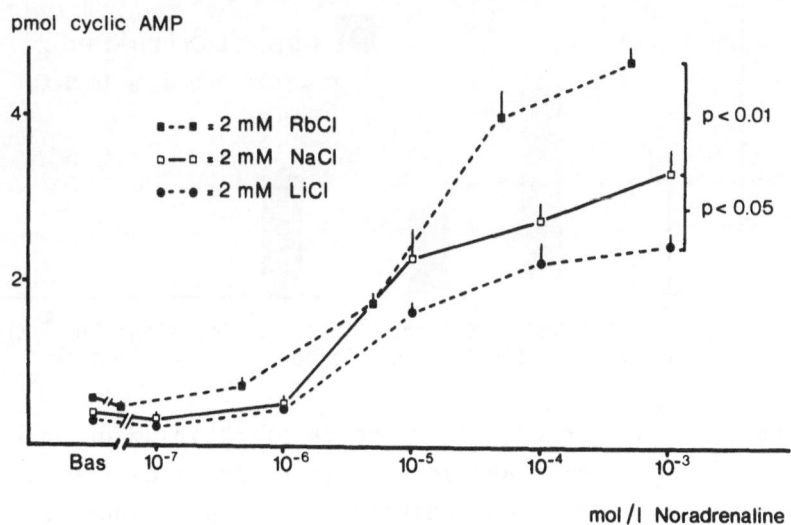

FIGURE 2   Effects of NaCl, RbCl and LiCl on noradrenaline-stimulated
            cyclic AMP accumulation in slices from rat cerebral cortex

Rubidium, on the other hand, enhanced in the same concentration the noradrenaline-stimulated cyclic AMP formation significantly ($p < 0.01$). It can also be seen in Figure 2 that
neither ion changed unstimulated adenylate cyclase activity.

In another experiment (Figure 3), using the same preparation
and identical experimental conditions, it was demonstrated
that the inhibitory effect of lithium and the enhancing effect of rubidium were neutralized or "antagonized" by the
combined addition of the two monovalent cations.

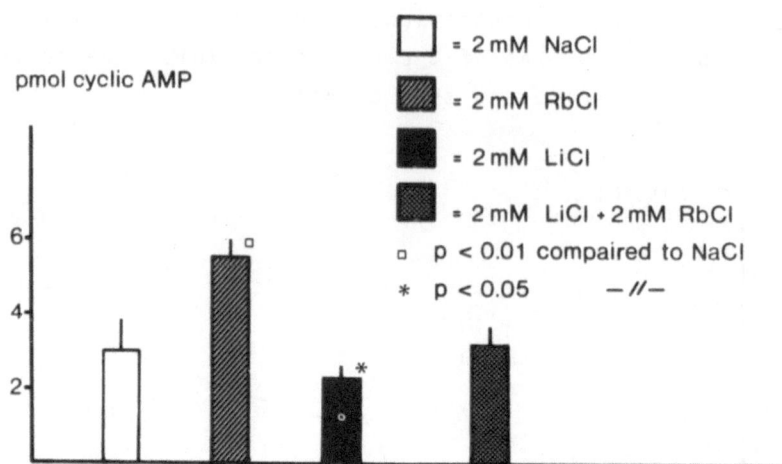

FIGURE 3   Effects of NaCl, LiCl and RbCl on noradrenaline (10^{-4} M)-
stimulated cyclic AMP accumulation in slices from rat
cerebral cortex

Further elucidation of the influence of rubidium on noradrenaline-induced cyclic AMP accumulation indicates that this
effect of rubidium is concentration-dependent, increases the
Vmax of the enzyme without altering the ED_{50}-value for noradrenaline, while basal enzyme activities, as mentioned, are
consistently unchanged.

In an additional study, using the same experimental conditions, we have compared the effect of potassium (2 mM) with
that of sodium in the same concentration and found that potassium, in this concentration, did not cause any changes
in noradrenaline-induced cyclic AMP accumulation.

4. Discussion.

Meaningful studies of the effects of lithium on those disturbances in the central nervous system involved in the
pathophysiology of affective disorders are hampered by the
lack of adequate animal models of mania and of depression.
Another problem in establishing relevant studies of the
mechanism of action of lithium is our limited understanding
or, in fact, ignorance of the psychobiological factors and

dysfunctions associated with clinical depression. The drugs we typically employ against depression or mania are not specific for any neurotransmitter and, in addition their acute effects which have been studied for so long may be quite different from their chronic effects. Thus, we are left with complicated research problems. However, clarification of and understanding of the mode of action of lithium may, due to its unique effect in the treatment of manic-depressive illness and related affective disorders, be the clue solving these apparently insoluble problems. Yet, despite an enormous volume of biochemical data, the site and the mode of action of lithium are still obscure. In fact, it is not clear whether observed neurochemical alterations are causal or consequential.

Various theories have been proposed. One states that lithium exerts its therapeutic effects by an interference with the noradrenaline-stimulated activity of cerebral adenylate cyclase. This hypothesis was initially based on the observations that lithium treatment reduced urinary cyclic AMP excretion in hypomanic patients and caused an increase in patients suffering from depression. However, a number of other studies on urinary cyclic AMP excretion and the cyclic AMP levels in cerebrospinal fluid from patients with affective disturbances have not confirmed a relation between mood disorders and the turnover and the function of cyclic AMP (36).

As discussed in Section 2, several studies have shown that lithium, undisputably, can inhibit some adenylate cyclases. Presently, it is most likely that this effect of lithium, at least in part, may explain some of the side effects of lithium, primarily polyuria (37), thyroid alterations (38), and possibly lithium-induced aggravation of psoriasis (39).

Proper interpretation of the clinical relevance and the ability of lithium to inhibit cerebral adenylate cyclase is not yet possible and any conclusion must still be considered speculative. First, the neurophysiological and psychological role of the beta-adrenergic cerebral adenylate cyclase is not understood. Secondly, it has become increasingly clear that the networks of noradrenergic neurones involved in synaptic transmission are intimately associated within the brain with serotonergic, cholinergic, dopaminergic, and other, so far, unknown transmitter systems. Thirdly, receptor-receptor interactions may exist in the central nervous system and represent an important synaptic integrative mechanism, e.g. the modulation of an aminergic receptor by a neuropeptide receptor. These, and other, circumstances presently prevent our understanding of the mechanisms by which lithium exerts its therapeutic actions.

However, the influence of lithium on adenylate cyclase is of considerable interest to researchers investigating this enzyme and its significance for synaptic transmission. This is the cause, because the interaction of lithium with adenylate cyclase is specific, i.e. the other monovalent cations sodium, potassium, caesium, and rubidium do not inhibit the activity of the enzyme, and furthermore selective, since only hormonal activation of the enzyme is affected. Therefore, lithium can be used as a tool in studies aiming at clarifying the processes that participate in hormone stimulation of adenylate cyclase.

As concluded in Section 2, lithium probably interferes with the transfer of the hormonal stimulus to the catalytic subunit. Our hypothesis is that lithium, as indicated in figure 4, inhibits the function of G/Fs dimer either by influencing the dissociation of the two components of the dimer or by interfering with a conformational change of the G/Fs protein itself.

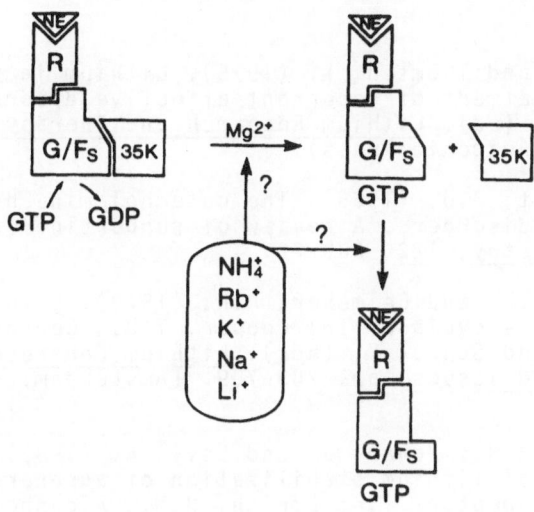

FIGURE 4   Schematic diagram of hypothetical influences of mono-
            valent cations on the G/Fs component. See text for
            explanation

In fact, we have recently observed that lithium in vitro
inhibits the stimulation of striatal adenylate cyclase by
the GTP analogue GDP(NH)P. It is still unknown if rubidium
possesses the opposite effect(s). Recently, Neer & Salter
have provided evidence that a monovalent cation, i.e. am-
monium sulphate, albeit in a high concentration, can facilitate the process depicted in Figure 4 (40).

While the clinical action of lithium is now well established, it is obvious that the pathogenesis of the affective
disorders and the mode of action of lithium are obscure.
Presumably, a number of strategies are necessary to un-
cover these enigmas. The influence of lithium and rubidium
on the noradrenaline-sensitive adenylate cyclase in brain
may be one of these strategies.

REFERENCES

1. Schou, M. and Thomsen, K. (1975). Lithium in the prophylactic treatment of recurrent affective disorders. In:
Johnson, F.N. (ed). Lithium Research and Therapy. pp. 63-
84. (London: Academic Press).

2. Schildkraut, J.J. (1965). The catecholamine hypothesis
of affective disorders. A review of supporting evidence.
Am. J. Psychiatry, 122, 509-22.

3. Ebstein, R.P. and Belmaker, R.H. (1979). Lithium and
brain adenylate cyclase. In: Cooper, T.B., Gershon, S.,
Kline, N.S. and Schou, M. (eds). Lithium Controversies
and Unresolved Issues. pp. 703-709. (Amsterdam: Excerpta
Medica).

4. Belmaker, R.H., Zohar, J. and Levy, A. (1982). Unidirectionality of lithium stabilization of adrenergic and
cholinergic receptors. In: Emrich, H.M., Aldenhoff, J.B.
and Lux, H.D. (eds). Basic Mechanisms in the Action of
Lithium. pp. 146-153. (Amsterdam: Excerpta Medica).

5. Sulser, F. (1982). Antidepressant drug research: Its
impact on neurobiology and psychobiology. In: Costa, E.
and Racagni, G. (eds). Advances in Biochemical Psychopharmacology, Vol. 31. pp. 1-20. (New York: Raven Press).

6. Goodwin, F.K., Ebert, M.H. and Bunney, W.E. (1972).
Mental effects of reserpine in man: a review. In: Shader,
R.I. (ed). Psychiatric Complications of Medical Drugs.
pp. 73-101. (New York: Raven Press).

7. Stolk, J.M., Conner, R.L. and Barchas, J.D. (1971).
Rubidium and lithium: evaluation as antidepressant and
antimanic agents. Psychopharmacologia (Berl.), 22, 250-60.

8. Paschalis, C., Jenner, F.A. and Lee, C.R. (1978).
Effects of rubidium chloride on the course of manic-depressive illness. J. Roy. Soc. Med. 71, 343-52.

9. Aurbach, G.D. (1982). Polypeptide and amine hormone
regulation of adenylate cyclase. In: Edelman, J.S. and
Berne, R.M. (eds). Ann. Rev. Physiol. 44, 653-66.

10. Rodbell, M. (1983). The complex structure and regulation of adenylate cyclase. In: Strange, P.G. (ed). Cell
Surface Receptors. pp. 228-239. (Chichester: Ellis Hor-
wood).

11. Geisler, A. and Klysner, R. (1978). Influence of lithium on dopamine-stimulated adenylate cyclase in rat
brain. Life Sci. 23, 635-6.

12. Wolff, J., Berens, S.C. and Jones, A.B. (1970). Inhibition of thyrotropin-stimulated adenyl cyclase activity of beef thyroid membranes by low concentration of lithium ion. Biochem. Biophys. Res. Commun. 39, 77-82.

13. Geisler, A. and Klysner, R. (in press). The effect of lithium in vitro and in vivo on dopamine-sensitive adenylate cyclase activity in rat brain homogenates. Acta pharmacol. et toxicol.

14. Shimizu, H., Ichishita, H. and Odagiri, H. (1974). Stimulated formation of cyclic adenosine 3',5'-monophosphate by aspartate and glutamate in cerebral cortical slices of guinea pig. J. Biol. Chem. 249, 5955-62.

15. Horn, A.S. and Phillipson, O.T. (1976). A noradrenaline-sensitive adenylate cyclase in the rat limbic forebrain: Preparation, properties and the effects of agonists, adrenolytics and neuroleptic drugs. Eur. J. Pharmacol. 37, 1-11.

16. Forn, J. and Valdecasas, F.G. (1971). Effects of lithium on brain adenylate cyclase activity. Biochem. Pharmacol. 20, 2773-8.

17. Schorderet, M. (1977). Lithium inhibition of cyclic AMP accumulation induced by dopamine in isolated retinae of the rabbit. Biochem. Pharmacol. 26, 167-70.

18. Geisler, A. and Klysner, R. To be published.

19. Gagnon, D.J. (1976). Lithium-angiotensin interaction in rat neurohypophysis. J. Cyclic Nucl. Res. 2, 251-6.

20. Ebstein, R.P., Hermoni, M. and Belmaker, R.H. (1980). The effect of lithium on noradrenaline-induced cyclic AMP accumulation in rat brain: Inhibition after chronic treatment and absence of supersensitivity. J. Pharmacol. Exp. Ther. 213, 161-7.

21. Hermoni, M., Lerer, B., Ebstein, R.P. and Belmaker, R.H. (1980). Chronic lithium prevents reserpine-induced supersensitivity of adenylate cyclase. J. Pharm. Pharmacol. 32, 510-1.

22. Murphy, D.L., Donelly, C. and Moskowitz, J. (1973). Inhibition by lithium of prostaglandin E_1 and norepinephrine effects of cyclic adenosine monophosphate production in human platelets. Clin. Pharmacol. Ther. 14, 810-4.

23. Friedman, E., Oleshansky, M.A., Moy, P. and Gershon, S. (1979). Lithium and catecholamine-induced plasma cyclic AMP elevation. In: Cooper, T.B., Gershon, S., Kline, N.S. and Schou, M. (eds). Lithium Controversies and Unresolved Issues.pp. 730-735. (Amsterdam: Excerpta Medica).

24. Ebstein, R., Belmaker, R., Grunhaus, L. and Rimon, R. (1976). Lithium inhibition of adrenaline-stimulated adenylate cyclase in humans. Nature,259, 411-3.

25. Geisler, A., Vendsborg, P.B., Johannesen, M., Klysner, R. and Thomsen, J. (1976). The effect of lithium on unstimulated and glucagon-stimulated urinary cyclic AMP excretion in rat and man. Acta pharmacol. et toxicol. 38, 433-9.

26. Sulser, F. (1983). Mode of action of antidepressant drugs. J. Clin. Psychiatry, 44, 5 (sec. 2), 14-20.

27. Pert, A. and Bunney, W.E. (1982). Chronic lithium modulates neurotransmitter receptor sensitivity. In: Emrich, H.M., Aldenhoff, J.B. and Lux, H.D. (eds). Basic Mechanisms in the Action of Lithium. pp. 121-132. (Amsterdam: Excerpta Medica).

28. Stolk, J.M., Nowack, W.J. and Barchas, J.D. (1970). Brain norepinephrine: enhanced turnover after rubidium treatment. Science, 168, 501-3.

29. Platman, S.R. (1971). Lithium and rubidium: A role in the affective disorders. Dis. nerv. Syst. 32, 604-6.

30. Meltzer, H.L., Taylor, R.M., Platman, S.R. and Fieve, R.R. (1969). Rubidium: A potential modifier of affect and behavior. Nature, 223, 321-2.

31. Tyrer, S. and Shopsin, B. (1980). Neural and neuromuscular side-effects of lithium. In: Johnson, F.N. (ed). Handbook of Lithium Therapy. pp. 279-309. (Lancaster: MTP Press).

32. Carroll, B.L. and Sharp, P.T. (1971). Rubidium and lithium: opposite effects on amine-mediated excitement. Science, 172, 1355-7.

33. Fieve, R.R. and Meltzer, H.L. (1974). Rubidium salts: Toxic effects in humans and clinical effects as an antidepressant drug. Psychopharmacol. Bull. 10, 38-50.

34. Personal communication.

35. Klysner, R., Geisler, A. and Andersen, P.H. (1983). Antidepressants and components of the beta-adrenoceptor system: Studies on zimelidine. In: Clinical Pharmacology in Psychiatry. 3rd International Meeting, Odense. (London: Macmillan Press). In press.

36. Geisler, A., Bech, P., Johannesen, M. and Rafaelsen, O.J. (1976). Cyclic AMP levels in cerebrospinal fluid in manic-melancholic patients. Neuropsychobiology, 2, 211-20.

37. Christensen, S. and Geisler, A. (1977). Antidiuretic and urinary cyclic AMP response of vasopressin in normal rats and in rats with lithium-polyuria. Acta pharmacol. et toxicol. 40, 44-54.

38. Männistö, P.T. (1980). Endocrine side-effects of lithium. In: Johnson, F.N. (ed). Handbook of Lithium Therapy. pp. 310-322. (Lancaster: MTP Press).

39. Bakker, B.J. and Pepplinkhuizen, L. (1980). Cutaneous side-effects of lithium. In: Johnson, F.N. (ed). Handbook of Lithium Therapy. pp. 372-377. (Lancaster, MTP Press).

40. Neer, E.J. and Salter, R.S. (1981). Reconstituted adenylate cyclase from bovine brain. J. Biol. Chem. 256, 12102-7.

5
The effect of rubidium and lithium on adenylate cyclase and neurotransmitter receptors

R. H. BELMAKER, R. HAMBURGER-BAR, M. NEWMAN AND J. BANNET

INTRODUCTION

This paper will compare lithium (Li) and rubidium (Rb) effects in the context of two current theories of Li action: 1) Inhibition of noradrenaline (NA)-sensitive adenylate cyclase, and 2) stabilization of receptor sensitivity changes induced by other treatments.

INHIBITION OF NA-SENSITIVE ADENYLATE CYCLASE

Inhibition of adenylate cyclase has been an attractive theory of Li action since Dousa and Hechter (1) first reported that Li can inhibit noradrenaline (NE)-sensitive adenylate cyclase in rat brain homogenates. When adenylate cyclase was proposed to be the second messenger for NE neurotransmission (2), Li inhibition of adenylate cyclase was easily related to an overall theory of affective disorder psychopharmacology: Schildkraut (3) proposed that NE neurotransmission is excessive in mania, Li is antimanic (4), and Li could be shown to inhibit second messenger function distal to the NE receptor (5).

However, this theory received a severe setback with the realization that Dousa and Hechter (1) and other early workers, had used high concentrations of Li to achieve adenylate cyclase inhibition. These concentrations could most likely be related to mechanisms of Li toxicity, rather than mechanism of Li action (6). Moreover, adenylate cyclase is a widely-spread enzyme in the body and in itself is nonspecific, the tissue specificity being determined by the receptor to which it is attached (7). Inhibition of adenylate cyclase therefore seemed to be a

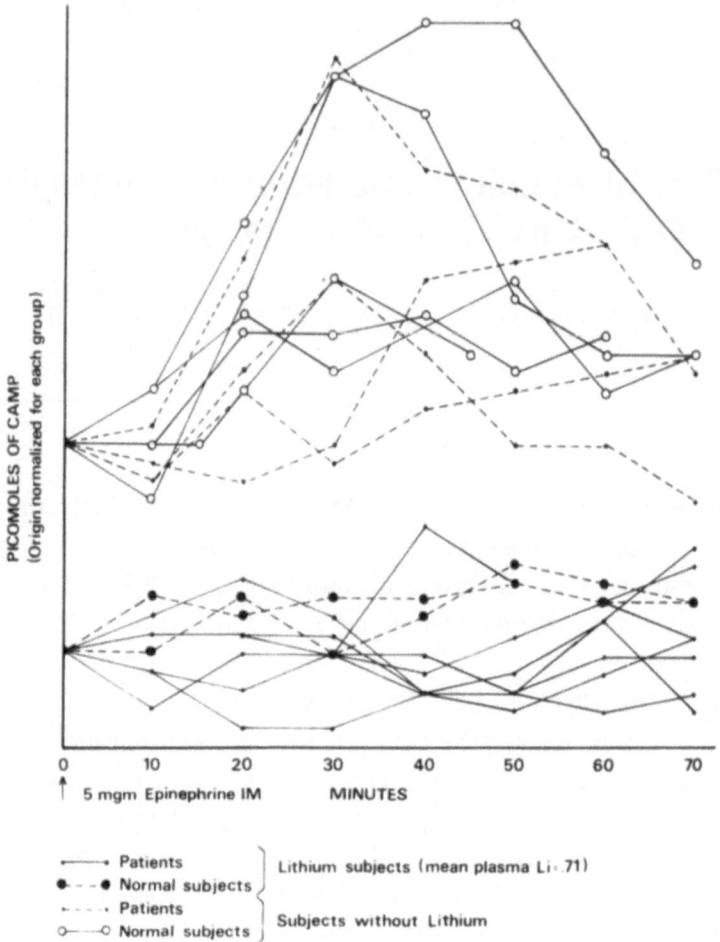

FIGURE 1   The effect of Li on plasma cyclic AMP response to adrenaline
administration. Subjects received 0.5 mg adrenaline subcuta-
neously at time 0 and blood was drawn every 10 min using an
indwelling catheter in the antecubital vein. (Subcutaneous
adrenaline injection was chosen rather than intravenous injection for greater clinical safety, in spite of the possibility of increased variability.) Samples were collected in plas-
tic test tubes containing heparin and theophylline. Cyclic
AMP was determined by the protein binding method.

All subjects were physically healthy consenting
adults. The lithium subjects (6 males, 3 females) had a mean
age of 38±3.6. Mean plasma lithium level was 0.71 mEq l^{-1}
with a range 0.32-1.15 mEq l^{-1}. The no-lithium control subjects (7 males, 1 female) had a mean age of 34±3.6. The lithium subjects included four manic-depressive patients and

fig. 1   one unipolar depressive patient, all in euthymic states; a
(cont.)   hypomanic manic-depressive patient; an euthymic schizo-
           affective patient; and two normal individuals. The no-lithium
           subjects included one euthymic manic-depressive patient; one
           depressed unipolar patient; one agitated schizo-affective
           patient; one hypomanic manic-depressive patient and five nor-
           mal inidividuals. Comparison (not shown) of the response of
           normal individuals without lithium to the response of patients
           without lithium does not suggest any effect of diagnosis or
           clinical state on the plasma cyclic AMP response to adrenaline.

more likely mechanism for the widespread symptoms of Li toxicity at
high Li concentrations, rather than the highly specific therapeutic
effects of Li at clinical concentrations. The concept that Li inhibition of adenylate cyclase could explain Li's antimanic action was put
aside as a misleading oversimplification almost as quickly as it had
previously become a leading theory.

In 1976 Ebstein et al (8) reported that patients on chronic Li
treatment had a markedly inhibited plasma cyclic AMP rise after epinephrine injection, compared with controls. The patients' Li levels were
nontoxic and well within the therapeutic range. Ball et al (9) had previously shown that the plasma cyclic AMP rise after epinephrine injection is due to stimulation of a peripheral β-adrenergic adenylate cyclase. At once it was clear that Li could inhibit adenylate cyclase in
vivo at therapeutic concentrations. Moreover, glucagon-induced rises in
plasma cyclic AMP in humans were then shown *not* to be inhibited in
patients receiving chronic Li treatment (10). Thus Li inhibition of
adenylate cyclase could be specific   because the adenylate
cyclase does differ in minor ways from tissue to tissue. Only minor
differences in Li sensitivity of adenylate cyclase would be required to
achieve specificity, as Li is a drug with a very narrow therapeutic
index. For instance, a "therapeutic target" adenylate cyclase might be
most sensitive to Li inhibition, which should occur in such a tissue
below 2.0mM Li. Other adenylate cyclases would need to be only slightly less sensitive to Li to be unaffected during clinical treatment
which is carried out carefully to remain below blood Li levels of 2.0mM.

A prime candidate for the target "adenylate cyclase" of Li treatment
is the NE-sensitive adenylate cyclase, which appears to be inhibited at
lower concentrations than the dopamine-sensitive adenylate cyclase (11),

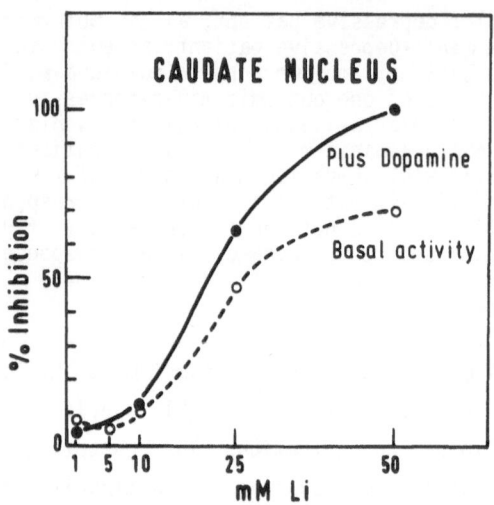

FIGURE 2   Inhibition by Li at high concentrations of the DA-sensitive
adenylate cyclase. Lithium inhibition of cell-free DA-
sensitive adenylate cyclase from mouse (C57 B1) caudate
nucleus reaches significance only at high (10-25 mM) concentrations. Mouse enzyme was used since we found it to be significantly more active than the rat DA-sensitive cyclase
although both species showed similar insensitivity to the
inhibitory action of Li. The tissue was homogenized in 50
volumes of 2 mM Tris-maleate buffer, pH 7.3, containing 1
mM EGTA. Ten μl of the tissue suspension was incubated for
2.5 minutes at 30°C with 40 μl of medium containing the
following components: 5 μCi of ^{3}H ATP, (2-^{3}H) adenosine 5'-
triphosphate (Amersham) diluted to a final concentration of
0.1 mM with non-radioactive ATP (the triated ATP was routine-
ly purified by Dowex 1 chromatography to ensure low blank
values); 80 mM Tris-maleate buffer, pH 7.3; 5 mM $MgSO_4$; 10
mM theophylline, and 0.15 mM cyclic AMP; 2.5 μg phosphatidyl
inositol, and 10 μM 5' guanylyl-imidodiphosphate. The concentration of DA was 100 μM. The reaction was stopped by
boiling and the cyclic AMP separated from the ^{3}H-ATP by
Dowex 50 chromatography. The percent stimulation above basal
activity averaged 100%. (From ref. #15.)

the parathormone-sensitive adenylate cyclase (12), or the glucagon-sensitive adenylate cyclase (10). Some adenylate cyclases such as the TSH-sensitive adenylate cyclase (13) and the ADH sensitive cyclase (14), are inhibited by Li, perhpas to a lesser degree than the NE-sensitive adenylate cyclase, but enough to relate to Li side effects on the kidney and thyroid (15,16). Some adenylate cyclases have not yet been studied for Li effects, such as the serotonin-sensitive adenylate cyclase (17). Preliminary work on the adenosine-sensitive adenylate cyclase suggests that it is sensitive to Li inhibition at 1.0mM Li (18).

Recent experimental work suggests that adenylate cyclase assays in cell-free homogenates are much less sensitive to Li inhibition than tissue slice assays containing whole cells (19). This explains the need for such high Li concentrations in the earliest work on Li and adenylate cyclase. A recent study (20) of Li effects on NE-sensitive adenylate cyclase in rat cortical tissue slices found clear Li inhibition in vitro by 2.0mM. The isoproterenol-induced cyclic AMP accumulation in the same study was significantly inhibited by 1.0mM Li. Chronic treatment of rats with Li leading to plasma levels of 1.73mM and ex vivo examination of NE-stimulated cyclic AMP accumulation showed a significant inhibition (20). Plasma levels of 1.73 mM are higher than the levels usual in psychiatric clinical practice today. Critics of the adenylate cyclase theory of Li action have suggested that these levels, low as they are, still represent the beginning of Li toxicity.

However, human cortex contains a NE-sensitive adenylate cyclase system that is several fold more active than that of the rat. That is, maximal rises of cyclic AMP are 12-40 fold over basal in human cortex (23,24) compared with 2-20 fold increases in rats (25). Such a more active system could well be more sensitive to Li inhibition. We recently were able to examine Li effects on NE-sensitive adenylate cyclase in human brain tissue obtained from the edges of surgically removed brain tumors. The brain tumors were sent to pathology where the healthy tissue was separated from tumor and then assayed for NE-sensitive adenylate cyclase activity within 8 hours after operation. Table 1 illustrates the results in 7 experiments on 7 fresh individual human brain samples, 6 frontal cortical grey matter and one temporal cortical grey matter.

Table 1.   Effect of Li on noradrenaline-stimulated cyclic AMP levels in incubated slices of human brain

	cAMP, pmol/mg protein
Control	106.7 ± 41.1
Noradrenaline, 50 uM	413.7 ± 77.5
Na, 50 μM + 0.5 mM Li	375.1 ± 93.8
NA, 50 μM + 1 mM Li	307.4 ± 74.3*
NA, 50 μM + 2 mM Li	327.9 ± 72.5**
NA, 50 μM + 5 mM Li	241.1 ± 65.5**

 * $p<0.05$, paired t-test compared with NA alone.
** $p<0.02$, paired t-test compared with NA alone.

These results strongly suggest that inhibition of noradrenaline-sensitive adenylate cyclase does take place at therapeutic concentrations of Li in human brain.

Table 2 shows the effect of 2mM and 5mM Rb on cyclic AMP accumulation in rat cortical slices, as used for Li (20). No inhibition of adenylate cyclase was demonstrated. There was a significant increase in basal accumulation in the absence of NA at 2mM Rb but not at 5mM Rb. There was a nonsignificant trend for an increase in the NA-induced rise at 5mM Rb only. This contrasts with data recently reported by Klysner and Geissler (this volume). However, Rb accumulates slowly in cells and preincubation times may be a critical factor. Our experiments, done without long preincubation with Rb, may not have allowed high enough concentrations of Rb to develop inside cells.

STABILIZATION OF RECEPTOR CHANGES INDUCED BY OTHER TREATMENTS
Pert et al (26) first reported that chronic Li prevents the increase in dopamine (DA) receptor sensitivity caused by three weeks of haloperidol feeding. They found this stabilization whether the DA receptor was measured biochemically or behaviorally. Others, however, have not been able to replicate the biochemical DA receptor stabilization and have found weak prevention of behavioral DA receptor sensitivity (27).

The effect of Li alone on DA receptors has also been a matter of controversy (28). While most authors find that Li induced no consistent change in DA receptor function, some groups have reported that in the period of Li withdrawal DA receptor number in the caudate is reduced (28,29).

Table 2. The effect of in vitro Rb on NA-induced increases in cyclic AMP accumulation

| | EXPERIMENT DAY | | | | | | | | | | | | | |
	I	II	III	IV	V	VI	VII	VIII	IX	X	XI	XII	XIII	x̄±SEM
control	1.1	1.4	3.6	2.1	2.3	0.7	1.5	2.0	2.9	2.4	1.0	2.6	2.0	2.03±.21
NA 50 μM	6.2	4.0	16.8	4.7	3.4	5.7	8.1	10.8	6.5	6.4	3.3	7.2	6.5	6.89±.99
Rb 2 mM	2.5	0.3	5.3	1.8	2.2	5.6	1.6	5.6	8.4	2.7	6.5	6.9	2.4	3.98±.69*
Rb 2mM + NA 50 μM	5.7	2.5	14.2	4.7	6.2	8.7	6.6	17.8	22.1	6.3	7.8	5.6	5.0	8.71±1.59
Rb 5 mM	-	1.3	4.3	1.6	1.0	2.4	1.8	4.2	10.2	2.2	1.1	2.2	3.3	2.96±0.73
Rb 5 mM + NA 50 μM	8.6	5.0	17.0	6.6	3.5	13.8	9.2	45.1	8.7	6.4	6.1	4.4	5.3	10.75±3.05

Cortical slices (1 mm cubes) were prepared using a McIlwain Tissue Chopper. The tissue was incubated in Krebs Ringer Bicarbonate solution containing glucose with continuous gassing (95% O_2 and 5% CO_2). After a 40 minute pre-incubation, the Ringer solution was changed and the tissue incubated for an additional 30 minutes in medium with and without RbCl. At the end of the second incubation period NA was added for an additional 6 minutes. The reaction was stopped by quickly collecting the tissue by filtration and rinsing with boiling distilled water (2 minutes). The tissue was then homogenized in 1 cc water and the cyclic AMP assayed using a kit supplied by the Radiochemical Center (Amersham, England). (From ref. #20)
* $p < .05$, paired t-test.

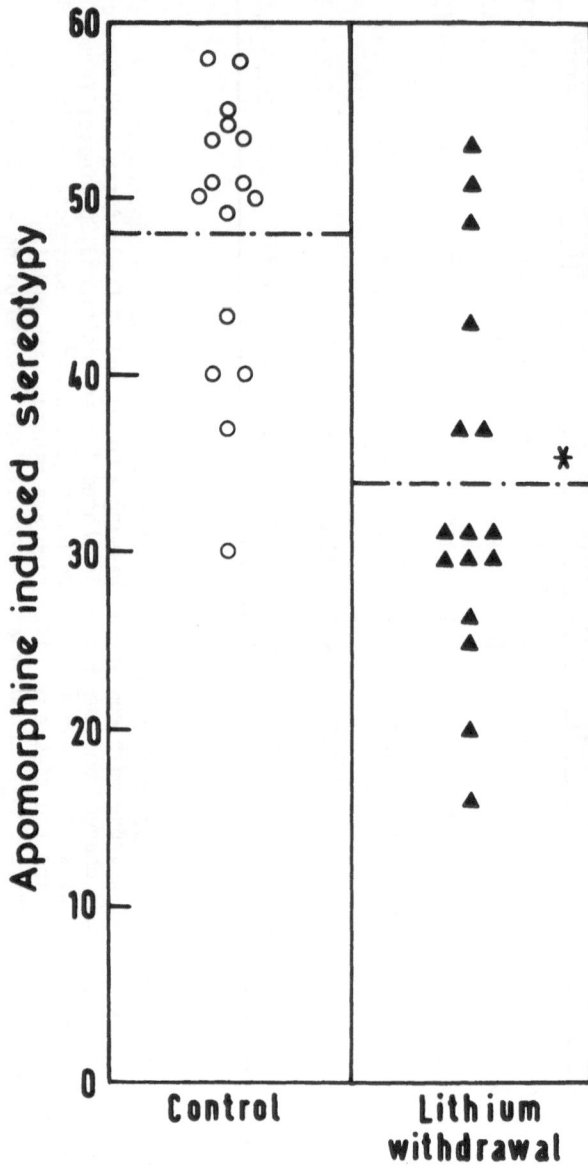

FIGURE 3   Stereotypy induced by apomorphine 2.5 mg/kg i.p. in rats
withdrawn for 48 hours after three weeks of chronic oral
lithium. Scale of Kelly and Iversen. (From ref. #31.)
* p<0.001

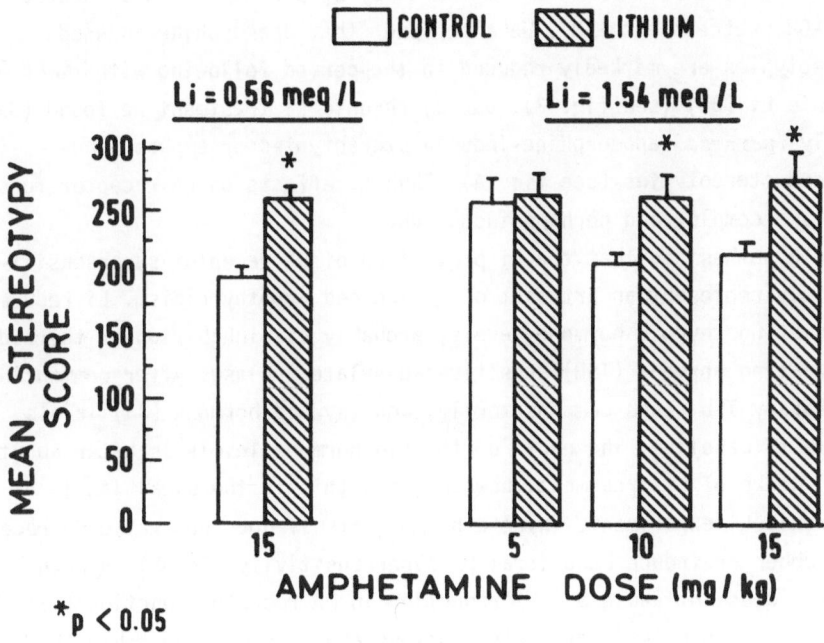

FIGURE 4   The effect of chronic Li on amphetamine-induced stereotypy.
Sabra strain (Hadassah) rats weighing approximately 150-200 g
were used in all experiments. Animals were maintained at 23±1
°C on a 12 h light-dark cycle. Li was ground up together with
standard rat pellets (either 0.1% or 0.2% Li per kg pellets)
and provided as a powder *ad lib* to the animals. The control
group received a similar diet except that Li was replaced by
sodium. At the end of 21-25 days of Li treatment separate
groups of rats (eight rats per group) were given i.p. 5, 10,
or 15 mg kg[-1] *d*-amphetamine sulfate dissolved in saline 25
min before stereotypy was measured (for a 15 min period) according to a slightly modified scoring system as described by
Costall and Naylor (1973). The intensity of stereotypic behavior was rated on a scale of 0-3 and included five categories: sniffing, licking, biting, head movements, and circling
behavior. Immediately after the experiments the rats were de-
capitated and serum Li levels determined by flame photometry.
Results are expressed as mean ± S.E.M. (From ref. #32)

Our group has found, in agreement with Pert et al (26), that Li can prevent DA receptor increases measured by spiperone binding, induced by 6-OH pretreatment (30). We also find that apomorphine-induced stereotypies are markedly reduced in the period following withdrawal of chronic Li (31) (see fig. 3). *During* chronic Li treatment we found (32) mildly *increased* apomorphine-induced stereotypies or amphetamine-induced stereotypies (see fig. 4). Thus Li effects on DA receptor function are complex and perhaps inconstant.

We hypothesized that the Li prevention of DA receptor supersensitivity may represent an artefact of Li-induced hypothyroidism. Li reduces circulating thyroid hormone levels, probably via inhibition of thyroid stimulating hormone (TSH)-sensitive adenylate cyclase. After commencing Li therapy TSH rises compensatorily, and thyroid hormone (33) levels return to baseline. The nadir of thyroid hormone levels is after about two weeks of Li treatment, however, and this is the usual length of a chronic Li experiment. Thyroid hormone itself does not raise DA receptor number or induce behavioral DA supersensitivity (34,35). Hypothyroidism does not cause a   reduction in DA receptor function (36). However, thyroid is a permissive hormone and it seemed possible that mild lowering of thyroid hormone levels would prevent the protein synthesis necessary for development of haloperidol-induced DA receptor supersensitivity. To test this hypothesis, we studied the effect of adding thyroid hormone to Li-treated rats.

Male Sabra rats weighing approximately 150g each were divided into 7 groups. The groups were fed as follows:

Group 1. normal ground food

     2. haloperidol .02% in ground food

     3. LiCl .2% in ground food

     4. DL-thyroxine 300 μg in 1 liter water (each rat thereby received between 3-4 μg per 100g weight per day. This is considered a replacement dose of thyroid hormone that should not cause hyperthyroidism in a normal rat but will reverse hypothyroid symptoms in a thyroid deficient rat (37,38).

     5. haloperidol .02% + Li 0.2% in ground food

     6. Li .2% in ground food + thyroxine 300 μg/L of drinking water.

     7. Li .2% + haloperidol .02% in ground food + thyroxine 300 μg/L of drinking water.

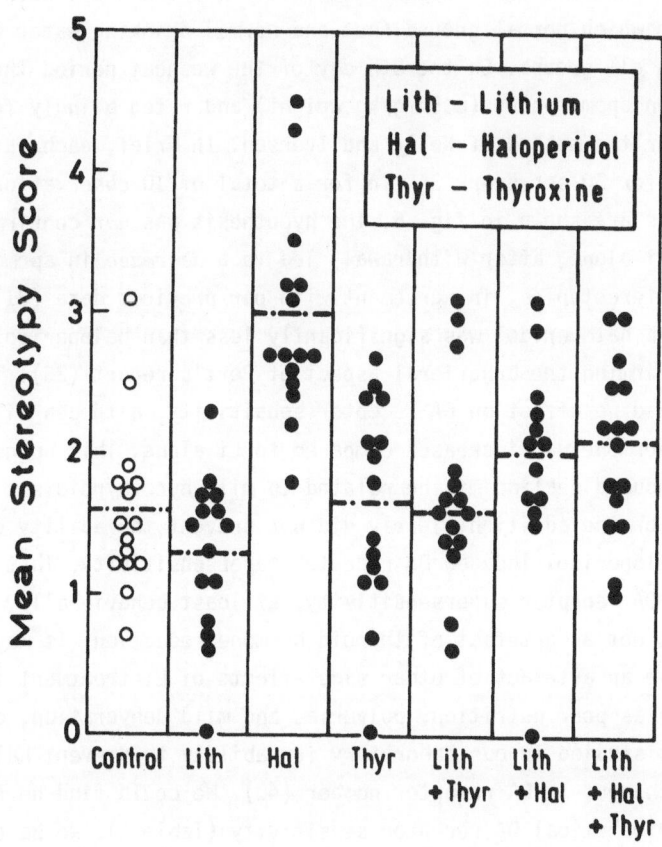

FIGURE 5   The effect of thyroid hormone on Li prevention of haloperidol-
induced subsensitivity. Haloperidol-treated group vs control,
t=5.2, p<.01. Li-treated vs controls, NS. Haloperidol-treated
vs Li+haloperidol, t=3.5, p<.01.

The groups receiving Li (#3,5,6,7) were started on Li 0.2% in ground food for 7 days. The other groups received normal ground food. After this 7-day period the haloperidol and thyroxine treatments were begun as described above for 4 weeks. Thereafter there was a 1 week washout period in which normal ground food and normal drinking water was administered to all groups. On the 8th day of the washout period the rats were given apomorphine (0.5 mg/kg weight) and rated blindly for stereotypy after the method of Kelly and Iversen. In brief, each rat was observed for 30 sec every 3½ min for a total of 10 observations.

Results are shown in fig. 5. The hypothesis was *not* confirmed. Chronic Li alone, after withdrawal, led to a *decrease* in apomorphine-induced stereotypies, in agreement with our previous data (31).

Li plus haloperidol was significantly less than haloperidol alone, thus confirming the behavioral aspect of Pert's report (26). Thyroid hormone had no effect on DA receptor sensitivity, although Li plus thyroid hormone was increased compared to Li alone. This suggests that the Li-induced decline may be related to mild hypothyroidism. However, thyroid hormone addition clearly did *not* prevent the ability of Li to reduce haloperidol-induced DA receptor supersensitivity. That is, Li prevents DA receptor supersensitivity, at least behaviorally, and this effect is not an artefact of thyroid hormone reduction. It may, of course, be an artefact of other side effects of Li treatment in the rat, such as poor nutrition, polyuria, and mild dehydration, etc. (39).

Rb was studied in our laboratory for ability to prevent haloperidol-induced changes in DA receptor number (40). We could find no Rb prevention of biochemical DA receptor sensitivity (Table 3). We have recently completed a study using behavioral techniques for measuring DA receptor function.

The results are shown in figure 6. Haloperidol leads as expected to significant behavioral DA receptor supersensitivity. Rb *also* causes such enhanced stereotypic responses to apomorphine as did Li (as discussed above, fig. 4). Rb plus haloperidol leads to less stereotypy than haloperidol alone or Rb alone. This decline is not statistically significant and in any case is difficult to interpret. It may be, however, that chronic Rb, like Li, interferes with the increase in behavioral sensitivity to DA agonists induced by chronic haloperidol. Thus haloperidol plus Rb is no different from Rb alone. This is unlikely to

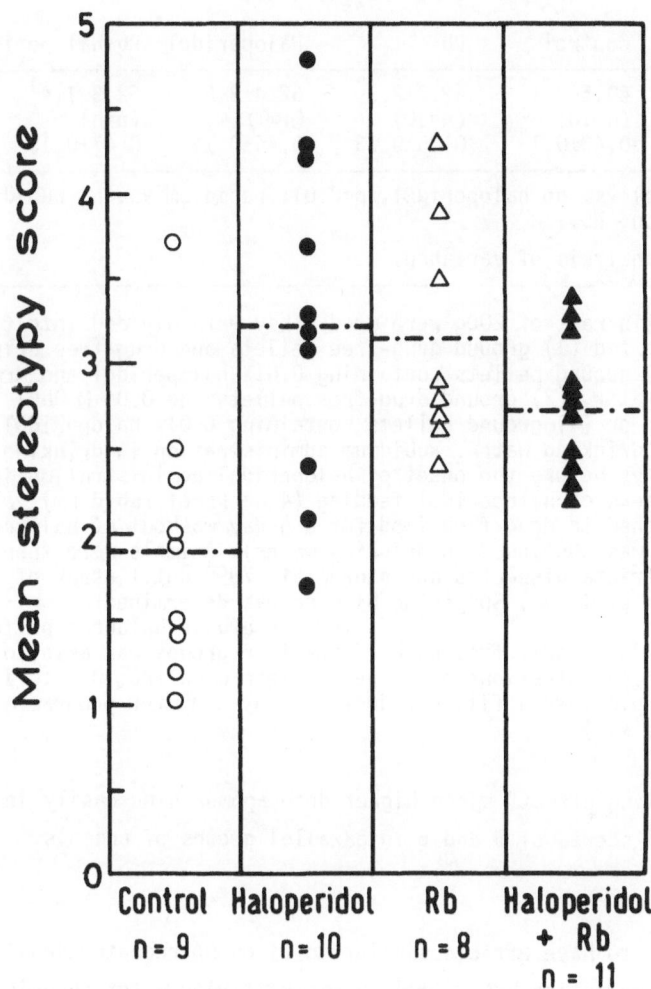

FIGURE 6   The effect of chronic oral rubidium treatment on haloperidol-
induced DA receptor   supersensitivity as measured by apomorphine-induced stereotypy. Chronic Rb and haloperidol feeding
as in Table 3. The same four-day washout was used, and then
animals were injected with apomorphine 1 mg/kg i.p. Animals
were observed for 30 seconds every 2 ⸢minutes for a total of
10 observations. Haloperidol-treated vs control, t=3.1,
p<.01. Rb vs haloperidol+Rb, NS. Rb-treated vs control, t=3.2,
p<.01. Rb treated animals showed no weight gain over the
course of the experiment while controls gained weight normally. The technical assistance of Ruth Kaso in this experiment
is gratefully acknowledged.

Table 3.   Effect of chronic rubidium on spiperone binding in rat
           caudate (pmol/g wet weight ± SD)

	Control	Rb	Haloperidol	Rb+haloperidol
Bmax	40.5±3.1 (n=10)	42.3±2.3 (n=10)	62.4±2.6 (n=9)	62.3±1.4[1] (n=8)
Kd, nM	0.43±0.1	0.35±0.13	0.44±0.14	0.47±0.15

Haloperidol vs. no haloperidol, p<0.01; rubidium vs. no rubidium, NS;
interaction, NS.

[1]Two-way analysis of variance.

Sabra strain rats of 200g were used. They were divided into four
groups and fed (1) ground drug-free pellets and drug-free drinking
water, (2) ground pellets containing 0.01% haloperidol and drug-free
drinking water, (3) ground drug-free pellets and 0.04 M RbCl in drinking water, or (4) ground pellets containing 0.01% haloperidol and 0.04M
RbCl in drinking water. Rubidium administration in drinking water was
begun 8 days before the onset of haloperidol administration in food.
After 3 weeks of haloperidol feeding (4 weeks of rubidium), all animals
were switched to drug-free food for a 4-day washout of haloperidol
(rubidium was continued in drinking water). Animals were then sacrificed
and the striata dissected and stored at -70°C until assay of spiperone
binding in striatum. Spiperone binding was determined
                              in a carefully balanced pattern in
which one individual from each of the four groups was assayed on each
day. Five concentrations of spiperone were used from 0.1 to 1 nM and
Scatchard plots were fitted objectively by computer programme.
(From ref. #40)

be a "ceiling effect" since higher dose apomorphine easily led to

stereotypy scores of 5 and 6 in parallel groups of animals.

SUMMARY

Rb appears to have effects similar to Li on DA receptor sensitivity

changes, preventing behavioral supersensitivity after chronic haloperi-

dol but not biochemical supersensitivity after chronic haloperidol.

Both Li and Rb when given chronically enhance apomorphine-induced

stereotypy. Li upon withdrawal leads to a subsensitivity to apomorphine;

Rb cannot be withdrawn acutely for the sake of comparison as its half-

life is too long.

    The effect of Li to prevent behavioral DA receptor supersensitivity

is not an artefact of Li-induced hypothyroidism. However, both the Li

and Rb effects may be due to poor nutrition or other factors that could

prevent behavioral supersensitivity after chronic haloperidol.

The effect of Li to inhibit adrenergic adenylate cyclase occurs at therapeutic Li concentrations in human periphery and in human brain. It is a highly replicable finding which may be related to Li's mode of action. Rb produces a tendency for an effect opposite to that of Li, that is, enhancement of noradrenaline-sensitive adenylate cyclase, but the Rb effect did not reach statistical significance.

REFERENCES

1. Dousa, T. and Hechter, O. (1970). Lithium and brain adenyl cyclase. *Lancet*, 834-835.
2. Robinson, G.A., Butcher, R.W. and Sutherland, E.W. (1971). *Cyclic AMP*. (New York: Academic Press)
3. Schildkrautt, J.J. (1965). The Catecholamine hypothesis of affective disorder. *Am. J. Psychiatry*, *122*, 509-522
4. Schou, M., Juel-Nielson, N., Stromgreen, E. and Volduy, H. (1954). The treatment of manic psychoses by the administration of lithium salts. *J. Neurol. Neurosurg. Psychiat.*, *17*, 250-260
5. Forn, J. and Valdecasas, F.G. (1971). Effects of lithium on brain adenyl cyclase activity. *Biochem. Pharmacol.*, *20*, 2773-2779
6. Belmaker, R.H. and Ebstein, R.P. (1979). Adenylate cyclase and the mechanism of lithium action. In: Saletu, B. (ed). *Neuropsychopharmacology*. pp. 95-101. (Oxford: Pergamon Press)
7. Nathanson, J.A. (1977). Cyclic nucleotides and nervous system function. *Physiological Reviews*, *57*, 157-255
8. Ebstein, R.P., Belmaker, R.H., Grunhaus, L. and Rimon, R. (1976). Lithium inhibition of adrenaline-sensitive adenylate cyclase in humans. *Nature*, *259*, 411-413
9. Ball, J.H. et al (1972). Effects of catecholamines and adrenergic blocking agents on plasma and urinary cyclic nucleotides in man. *J. Clin. Invest.*, *51*, 2124-2129.
10. Ebstein, R.P., Kara, T. and Belmaker, R.H. (1977). The effect of lithium on the glucagon-sensitive adenylate cyclase in vivo in man. *Acta Pharmacol. Toxicol.*, *41*, 0-83
11. Reches, A., Ebstein, R.P. and Belmaker, R.H. (1978). Differential effect of lithium on noradrenaline-and dopamine-sensitive accumulation of cyclic AMP in guinea pig brain. *Psychopharmacology*, *58*, 213-216

12. Spiegel, A.M. et al (1976). Lithium does not inhibit the parathy-
    roid hormone-mediate rise in urinary cyclic AMP and phosphate in
    humans. *J. Clin. Endocrinol. Metabol.*, *43*, 1390-1393

13. Wolff, J., Berens, S.C. and Jones, A.B. (1970). Inhibition of
    thyrotropin-stimulated adenyl cyclase activity of beef thyroid by
    low concentration of lithium ion. *Biochem. Biophys. Res. Comm.*,
    39, 77-83

14. Geisler, A., Wraae, O. and Olesen, O.V. (1972). Adenyl cyclase
    activity in kidneys of rats with lithium-induced polyuria. *Acta
    Pharmacol. Toxicol.*, *31*, 203-208

15. Ebstein, R.P. and Belmaker, R.H. (1979). Lithium and brain adenylate
    cyclase. In: Copper, T.B., Gershon, S., Kline, N.S. and Shou M.
    (eds). *Lithium Controversies and Unresolved Issues*. pp. 703-729.
    (Amsterdam: Experta Medica)

16. Ebstein, R.P. and Belmaker, R.H. (1977). A comparison of effect of
    lithium and haloperidol on human peripheral β-adrenergic adenylate
    cyclase. In: Gershon, E., Belmaker, R.H., Rosenbaum, M. and Kety,
    S. (eds). *The Impact of Biology on Modern Psychiatry*. (New York:
    Plenum Press)

17. Von Hungen, K., Roberts, S. and Hill, D.F. (1975). Serotonin-sen-
    sitive adenylate cyclase activity in immature rat brain. *Brain Res.*,
    84, 257-268

18. Ebstein, R.P., Reches, A. and Belmaker, R.H. (1978). Lithium inhi-
    bition of the adenosine-induced increase of adenylate cyclase acti-
    vity. *J. Pharm. Pharmac.*, *30*, 122-123.

19. Wang, Y.C., Pandey, G.N., Mendels, J. et al (1974). Effect of
    lithium on prostaglandin E 1-stimulated Adenylate cyclase activity
    of human platelets. *Biochem. Pharmacol.*, *23*, 845-855

20. Ebstein, R.P., Hermoni, M. and Belmaker, R.H. (1980). The effect of
    lithium on noradrenaline-induced cyclic AMP accumulation in rat
    brain: inhibition after chronic treatment and absence of supersen-
    sitivity. *J. of Pharmacol. and Experimental Therap.*, *213*, 161-167.

21. Noack, C.H. and Trautner, E.M. (1951). The lithium treatment of
    maniacal psychosis. *Med. J. Australia*, *38*, 219.

22. Klein, D.F., Gittelman, R., Quitkin, F. and Rifkin, A. (1980).
    *Diagnosis and Drug Treatment of Psychiatric Disorders: Adults and
    Children*. pp. 435-437. (Baltimore: Williams and Wilkins)

23. Fumagalli, R., Bernareggi, V., Berti, F. and Trabucchi, M. (1971). Cyclic AMP formation in human brain: an in vitro stimulation by neurotransmitters. *Life Sci.*, *10(I)*, 1111-1115

24. Shimizu, H., Tanaka, S., Suzuki, T. and Matsukado, Y. (1971). The response of human cerebrum adenyl cyclase to biogenic amines. *J. Neurochem.*, *18*, 1157-1161

25. Daly, J. (1977). *Cyclic Nucleotides in the Nervous System*. p. 130. (New York: Plenum Press)

26. Pert, A., Rosenblatt, J., Sivit, C., Pert C.B. and Bunney Jr., W.E. (1978). Long-term treatment with lithium prevents the development of dopamine receptor supersensitivity. *Science*, *201*, 171-173

27. Staunton, D.A., Magistretti, P.J., Shoemaker, W.J. and Bloom, F.E. (1982). Effect of chronic lithium on dopamine receptors in rat corpus striatum. *Brain Res.*, *232*, 391-400.

28. Pert, A. and Bunney Jr., W.E. (1982). Chronic lithium modulates neurotransmitter receptor sensitivity. In: Emrich, H.M., Aldenhoff, J.B. and Lux, H.D. (eds). *Basic Mechanisms in the Action of Lithium*. pp. 121-132. (Amsterdam: Excerpta Medica)

29. Kafak, M.S., Wirz-Justice, A., Naber, D., Marangos, P.J., O'Donahue, T.L. and Wehr, T.A. (1982). *Neuropsychobiology*, *8*, 41.

30. Eisenberg, J., Brecher-Fride, E., Weizman, R., Ebstein, R.P. and Belmaker, R.H. (1981). Lithium and receptors in rat model of MBD. In: Perris, C., Struwe, G. and Jansson, B. (eds). *Developments in Psychiatry*, *vol. 5 - Biological Psychiatry 1981*. (Amsterdam, Elsevier)

31. Lerer, B., Globus, M., Brik, E. and Hamburger, R. (1983). Effect of treatment and withdrawal from chronic lithium in rats on stimulant-induced responses. *Neuropsychobiology*, in press

32. Ebstein, R.P., Eliashar, S., Ben-Uriah, Y., Yehuda, S. and Belmaker R.H. (1980). Chronic lithium treatment and dopamine mediated behaviour. *Biological Psychiatry*, *15*, 459-467

33. Cooper, T.B. and Simpson, G.M. (1969). Preliminary report of a longitudinal study on the effect of lithium on iodine metabolism. *Curr. Therap. Res.*, *11*, 603-608

34. Atterwill, C.K. (1981). Effect of acute and chronic tri-iodothyronine (T_3) administration to rats on central 5-HT and dopamine-mediated behavioural responses and related brain biochemistry. *Neuropharmacology*, *20*, 131-144

6
Does lithium prevent the development of dopamine receptor supersensitivity? Behavioural studies

H. M. CALIL AND F. C. RODRIGUES

INTRODUCTION

Although lithium's efficacy in affective illness has been well proven (1), the mechanisms of action responsible for its therapeutic effect remain unknown, especially when one considers its long lasting dual antimanic and antidepressant properties. Several hypotheses have been formulated to explain how lithium exerts its action. Chronic lithium in clinically equivalent concentrations, inhibits differentially adenylate cyclases in animals and humans. Considering that these actions seem to be the most consistent findings of the lithium neurochemical studies, Belmaker and coworkers (2,3) suggested that it might be the mechanism of lithium action. Another hypothesis was raised by Bunney and coworkers. They first speculated that manic depressive illness might be caused, at least partially, by oscillations in catecholamine receptor sensitivity, in an attempt to further develop the original catecholamine hypothesis, thus extending it to the receptor level (4). Their idea was based on clinical observation that dopamine receptor antagonists (neuroleptics) acutely suppress manic symptomatology, while dopamine agonists (such as piribedil and l-Dopa) can precipitate manic episodes in certain depressed patients. These findings led to the idea that

77

receptor sensitivity changes underlie the behavioral signs in bipolar illness: mania being a consequence of an abnormal increase and depression from an abnormal decrease. Interestingly, this renewed interest in dopaminergic involvement in affective illness seems to parallel the appearance of drugs with potent dopamine inhibition effect and weak action on serotonergic and noradrenergic uptake systems, unlike the traditional tryciclic antidepressants, yet with therapeutic antidepressant properties. As a natural extension of this latter hypothesis, and since lithium is a powerful antimanic therapeutic agent, it was thought that it might prevent the development of dopamine receptor super sensitivity usually observed after long term treatment with neuroleptics. In fact, animal studies by Klawans (5,6) had already reported on a partial antagonism by lithium of the pharmacologically-induced dopamine behavioral super-sensitivity. These preliminary data were then followed by papers from Bunney's group showing the antagonism by lithium of the dopamine induced supersensitivity observed with behavioral (7); neurophysiological (8); and more interesting, neurochemical studies (9).

Several preclinical investigations, testing the hypothesis of lithium as a receptor stabilizer have been done in the last years. They were reviewed recently by Bunney and Garland (10). Most of the results show that lithium decreases the behavioral supersensitivity. This was not found on locomotor activity by Staunton and coworkers (11). Other groups found only a partial decrease of self-stimulation and an attenuation of stereotypy (11,12,13). Other ways of inducing dopaminergic supersensitivity have also been employed, namely the injection of 6-hydroxy-dopamine (14) and chronic reserpine (15). These latter studies found that lithium caused only partial decrease (14), or unexpectedly an increase of the behavioral super-sensitivity (15). Using ovariectomy as yet another method of inducing dopaminergic supersensitivity, lithium was able to cause a partial decrease of stereotypy (16).

In most of the above mentioned studies different tests were utilized to measure supersensitivity such as stereotypy, locomotor activity, aggressiveness, intracerebral self-stimulation and rotational behavior. Besides these, lithium was also studied in the test of catalepsy induced by haloperidol, and prevented the tolerance normally observed (supersensitivity) (17).

Great enthusiasm followed Bunney's group hypothesis, especially the animal data showing that lithium could stabilize receptor oscillations by preventing the proliferation of receptor sites after long term treatment with haloperidol. However, this biochemical effect of lithium has not been replicated by other groups (18,19,20). Lithium failed to prevent the receptor supersensitivity induced either by chronic treatment with haloperidol, or nigrostriatal lesion with 6-hydroxydopamine. It would be interesting to note that chronic lithium per se does not change (7) or may decrease the number of dopamine receptor sites (9,21,22).

Most of the mentioned studies utilized chronic lithium administration concomitant with the other supersensitivity inducing treatments. It was usually given with food, in the regular chow containing 0.2% of lithium. This lithium diet produces reliable serum levels, in the human clinical range, without any gross toxicity.

We have been interested for many years, in rapid eye movement (REM) sleep deprivation of animals as yet another way of supposedly inducing dopamine receptor supersensitivity. It has been shown by a number of investigators that selective REM sleep deprivation of rats is followed by an increased response to dopamine agonists stimulation. In our laboratory it has been measured by the stereotyped behavior induced by apomorphine or more typically by the aggressiveness elicited by larger doses of apomorphine (23,24). The method used to REM sleep deprivation of the animal has been called the flower pot technique (25), and consists of placing the rats on small platforms (7 cm in diameter) surrounded by water in a metal container. Food and water are provided ad libitum. In order to control this stressful manipulation, and perhaps for the isolation stress, an experimental control group is run simultaneously. The rats are then placed on larger platforms, that is, on top off an inverted flower pot of 14 cm in diameter. This allows REM sleep without the rats falling in the water. The results described with apomorphine were later extended to other dopamine agonists following different amounts of REM sleep deprivation (26). Carlini and coworkers decided to run a pilot study a few years ago to find out whether chronic lithium could also prevent the development of the behavioral supersensitivity seen after REM sleep deprivation. Groups of rats were fed a lithium diet for three weeks, one group was deprived of REM sleep during 96 h, another group was treated with haloperidol 1 mg/kg also for three weeks, and yet another with an association of haloperidol and lithium. When tested for aggressiveness it was found that lithium did not prevent the aggressive behavior induced by large dose apomorphine after REM sleep deprivation, and the pretreatment with haloperidol did not induce apomorphine elicited aggression on its withdrawal. These results were very discouraging, and never published.

However, as more evidence accumulated suggesting that REM sleep deprivation does induce behavioral dopaminergic super sensitivity, and at the same time lithium's ability of preventing the development of supersensitivity was questioned, we decided to undertake a systematic study.

STUDIES WITH CHRONIC NEUROLEPTIC

The first step was an attempt to replicate data previously described in the literature. We used four groups of 20 male Wistar rats, 3 to 4 months old, kept in an air-conditioned room (temperature: $24\pm1^{\circ}C$) with a 12 h light-dark cycle. They were treated with saline (control), haloperidol (1 mg/kg) intraperitoneal (I.P.), and the association of haloperidol (I.P.) and lithium (0.2%, added to the food),

during three weeks, Their mean weight was 292 g, ranging
from 250 to 350 g at the beginning of the experiment,without
differences of mean weight among the groups. Like Staunton
and coworkers (11), we also noticed no weight gain in the
lithium treated rats, whereas the others continued gaining
weight. Then, to control for this weight variable, partial
food deprivation was introduced on days 14 and 15 of chronic
treatment for the control and haloperidol groups. At the
end of 3 weeks of treatment, the weight variation was 6%
for the saline (control) group, 4.7% for haloperidol group,
1.6% for lithium group, and -2.6% for haloperidol + lithium
group. The lithium treated animals developed lithium serum
levels averaging $0.96^{\pm}0.26$, and ranging from 0.7 to 1.4
mEq/l. After withdrawing the three weeks treatment, they
were tested for catalepsy induced by haloperidol, stereotypy
and aggressiveness induced by different doses of apomorphine.

The catalepsy test was performed on the 5th day of chronic
treatment withdrawal, after injecting haloperidol 1 mg/kg.
The total observation time was 4 h, divided in 20 min
intervals, and starting 20 min after injection. The time the
rats remained in an upright position with the forepaws
resting on a glass bar was measured. Although there were
significant decreases in the first observation intervals for
the lithium and the association of haloperidol with lithium
pretreated groups as compared to the control group, the
differences disappeared when the total catalepsy time was
considered (Figure 1). The haloperidol pretreated group only
tended to show a decrease (tolerance) of catalepsy, and if
anything lithium concomitant to haloperidol pretreatment
appeared to potentiate the haloperidol decrease.

The stereotypy test was done on the 9th day of chronic
treatment withdrawal. Time and scores of stereotyped
behavior were measured for 5 min each time (a total 5
observation intervals) up to 60 min after injecting
apomorphine 0.6 mg/kg. The degree of stereotyped behavior
was rated on a 0 to 4 scale (27). The results show that
haloperidol pretreatment induced a significant increase of

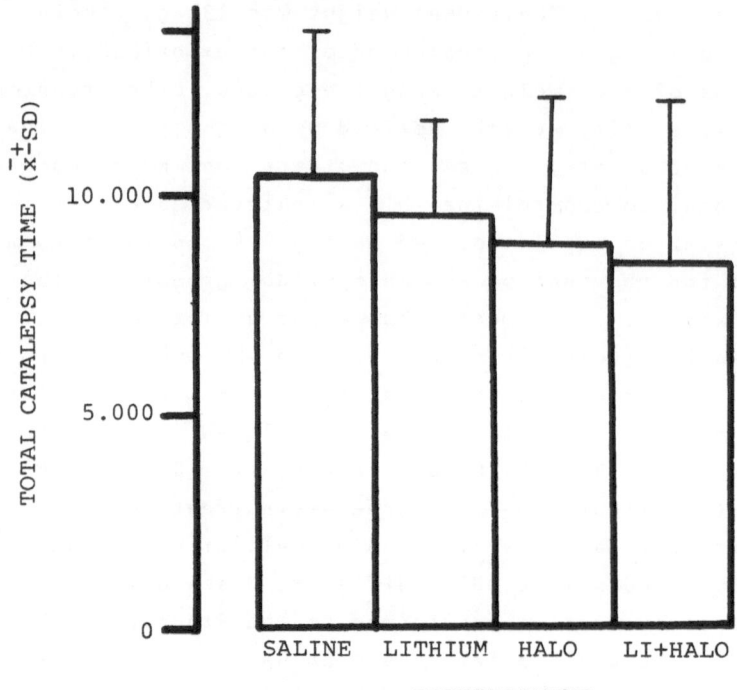

FIGURE 1   Mean total catalepsy time (sec) induced by haloperidol
(1 mg/kg, I.P.), on the 5th day withdrawal of chronic
pretreatment. N=10 for each group. Anova: N.S.
Abbreviations: haloperidol=HALO, lithium=LI.

stereotyped behavior time in several observation intervals.
However, the pretreatment with the association of haloperidol
+ lithium induced an even larger and significant increase
of stereotypy as compared to the control group. These
differences also were seen for the total stereotypy time
(Figure 2). Considering the stereotypy scores (Figure 3),
the increase observed in the haloperidol pretreated group
was not prevented by associating lithium to haloperidol
during the three weeks pretreatment, thus following the
same pattern observed with the total stereotypy time.

The test for aggressiveness was performed on the 14th day
withdrawal. The rats were injected with apomorphine 5 mg/kg
I.P., paired in wire cages, and the fighting time measured.
There were no significant differences among the groups,

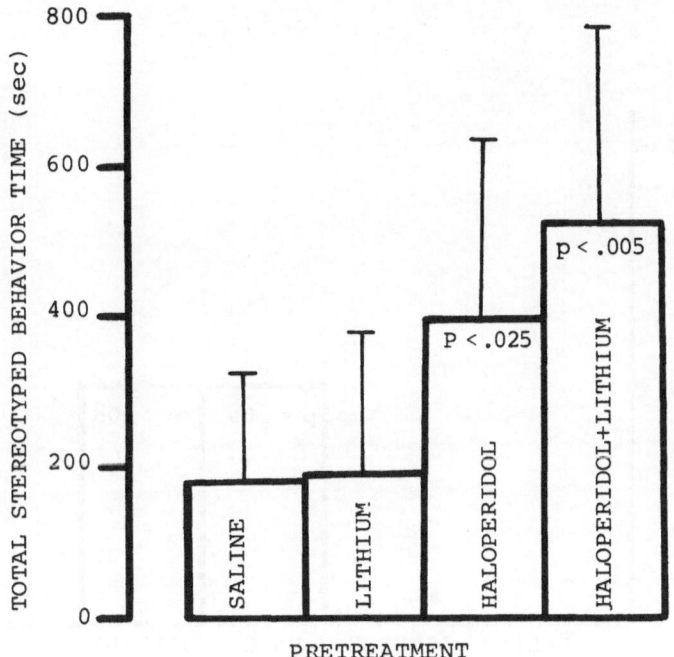

FIGURE 2   Stereotypy time ($\bar{x} \pm$SD) induced by apomorphine (0.6 mg/kg, I.P.) on the 9th day withdrawal of chronic pretreatment. N=10 for each group. Anova: p<0.005. The groups were compared to control (t-test), and p values are on the figure.

with a tendency for the lithium pretreated group to fight more, followed by the haloperidol pretreated group. This experiment was then run with another group of rats, similarly pretreated, but tested on the 5th day withdrawal. The results showed basically the same pattern, with the association of lithium and haloperidol pretreatment only tending to prevent the increased aggressiveness seen in the haloperidol pretreated group. Again the lithium pretreated group had a higher total aggressiveness time, but only one pair fought and the result was not significant.

STUDIES WITH REM SLEEP DEPRIVATION

The REM sleep deprivation was achieved with the method

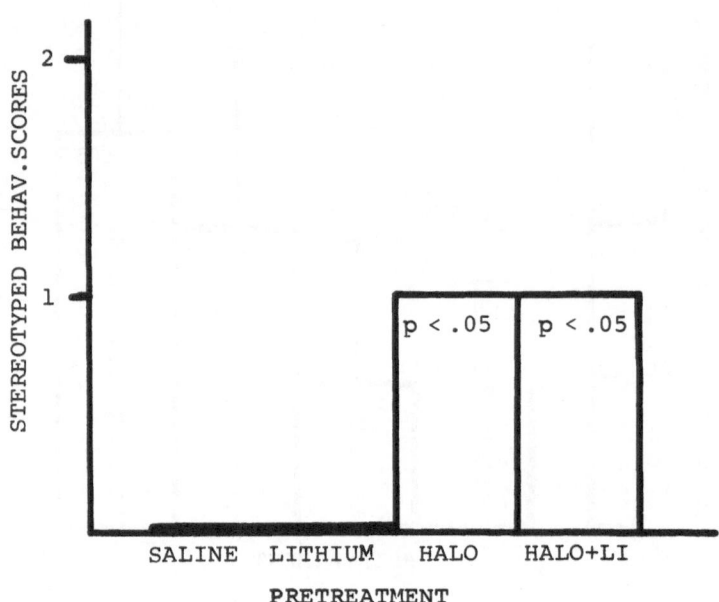

FIGURE 3   Scores of stereotypy induced by apomorphine (0.6 mg/kg
            I.P.) on the 9th day withdrawal of chronic pre-
            treatment. N=10 for each group. Kruskal-Wallis: p<0.05.
            Groups were compared to control (t-test), and p values
            are on the figure.

previously described. The same tests were done following
three weeks pretreatment with lithium or saline (control)
and REM sleep deprivation during 96 h. Both groups, the
experimental control (large platforms) and the REM sleep
deprived (small platforms) tended to have a tolerance to
catalepsy induced by haloperidol, whereas the lithium pretreated, as well as the lithium pretreatment and REM sleep
deprived groups, were almost identical to the control
group. In any case, only tendencies were seen since no
significant differences were found. This test was repeated
maintaining the lithium treatment during the 96 h of REM
sleep deprivation. Then, the total catalepsy time was
significantly increased by lithium alone and lithium

treatment + experimental control, whereas lithium treatment plus REM sleep deprivation did not pratically differ either from the control or the REM sleep deprived groups (Figure 4). These results confirm previous reported data (28) showing a potentiation by chronic lithium treatment of dopamine mediated behavior.

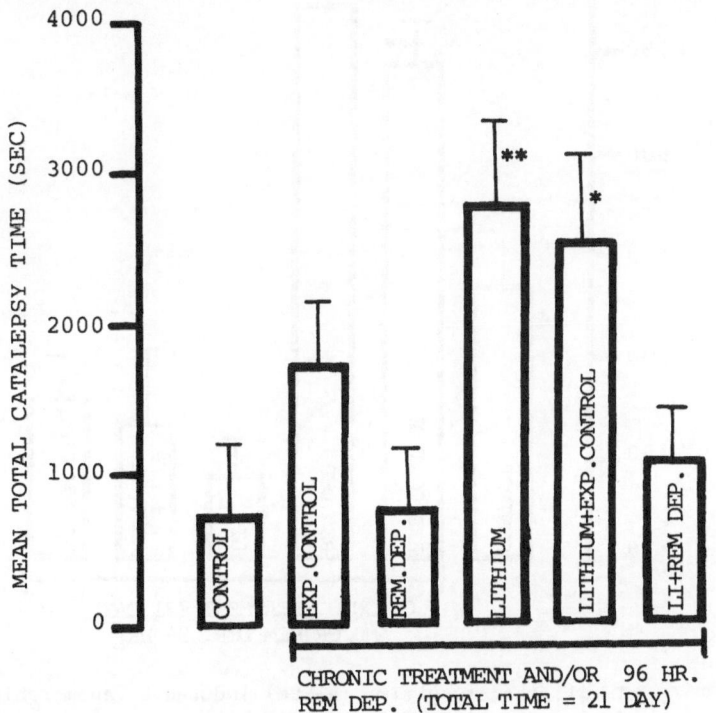

FIGURE 4   Catalepsy time ($\pm$ SEM) induced by haloperidol (1 mg/kg, I.P.). Anova: $p < .01$; t-test: $*p < .05$; $**p < .01$, compared to control group.

In the stereotypy test (apomorphine 0.6 mg/kg), both the experimental control and the REM sleep deprivation groups showed an increased stereotyped behavior time. The lithium pretreated group had a significant decrease of stereotypy time and lithium pretreatment prevented the increased response to apomorphine seen in both the REM sleep deprivation and experimental control groups (Figure 5). Pratically the same results were obtained for the stereotypy scores, except that in this case the lithium group did not differ from the control group, and it was clear that lithium pretreatment prevented the increased response to apomorphine.

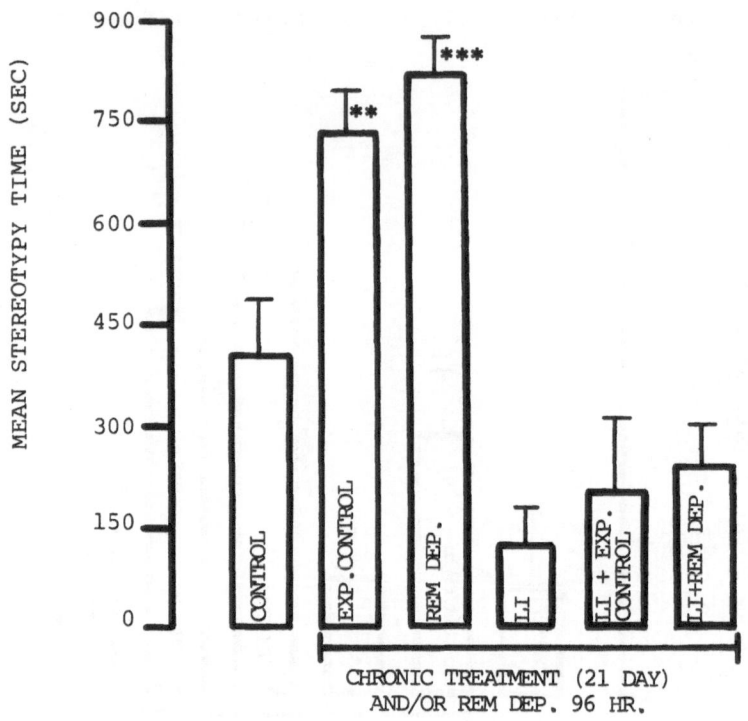

FIGURE 5   Total stereotypy time ($\bar{x} \pm$ SEM) induced by apomorphine (0.6 mg/kg, I.P.). Anova: $p < .001$; t-test (two-tailed): *$p < .02$; **$p < .01$; ***$p < .001$, compared to control group.

In the aggressiveness test, the experimental control and REM sleep deprivation groups showed significant increases of aggression time compared to control group. The lithium pretreated group did not differ from control, and lithium pretreatment followed by experimental control or REM sleep deprivation decrease the effects of these manipulations (Figure 6).

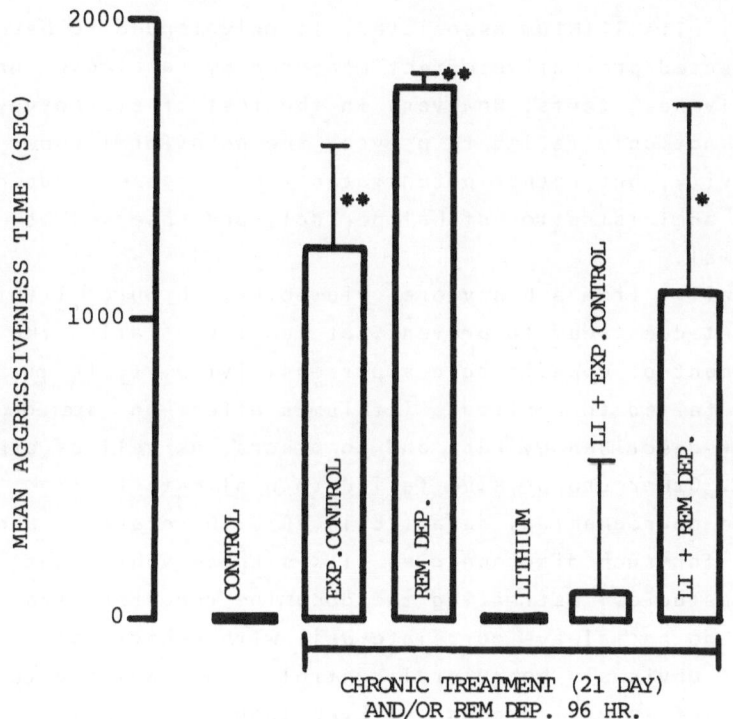

FIGURE 6   Total aggressiveness time ($\bar{x}\pm$SD) induced by apomorphine
(5 mg/kg, I.P.). Anova: p<.001; t-test (one-tailed):
*p<.005; **p<.0005, compared to control group.

SUMMARY AND CONCLUSIONS

Lithium pretreatment had the expected effect, that is, it
prevented the development of behavioral dopaminergic supersensitivity induced by REM sleep deprivation as measured
by stereotypy and aggressiveness tests. In both tests the
expected increase of response to apomorphine (supersensitivity) was seen in the REM sleep deprivation group.
However, the experimental control group also had
significant increase of stereotypy and aggressiveness. This
fact seems to implicate the "stress" inherent to the REM
sleep deprivation procedure inducing supersensitivity. It
was even further studied and discussed before (29). When
chronic haloperidol was the behavioral supersensitivity

inducer, with lithium associated, it only tended to have the expected preventive effect measured by catalepsy and aggressiveness tests. However, in the test of stereotypy lithium not only failed to prevent the behavioral supersensitivity, but rather potentiated the increase induced by chronic administration of haloperidol, and observed at withdrawal.

Generally, from a behavioral viewpoint, chronic lithium treatment does seem to prevent, at least partially, the development of dopaminergic supersensitivity. It is puzzling that we failed to replicate lithium's effect on stereotyped behavior described by Pert and coworkers, as well as other authors. Other groups also failed to duplicate their reported neurochemical data (18,19,20). There are no known reasons for such discrepancies. It is conceivable that binding studies, estimating the dopamine receptor site numbers do not always correlate well with behavioral studies. Obviously behavioral control is a final and complex endpoint of several processes. Even though the tests employed evaluate behavior with predominantly dopaminergic control, it is not possible to exclude the influence of other neurotransmitter systems, which are also modified by chronic lithium treatment (19,30,31). More work is needed to clarify the issue of lithium's prevention of receptor supersensitivity, before accepting the idea that lithium acts as a stabilizer of receptor sensitivity oscillations. Furthermore, this hypothesis which might predict that lithium should also inhibit the development of catecholamine receptor subsensitivity has not been supported by a number of experimental studies (32,33,34).

ACKNOWLEDGEMENT

Our gratitude to Ms.Ines Monaco for typing the manuscript. Work partially funded by CNPq and CAPES.

REFERENCES

1. Schou, M. and Thomsen, K. (1975). Lithium prophylaxis of recurrent endogenous affective disorders. In: Johnson, F. N. (ed). Lithium Research and Therapy. pp. 63-84. (London: Academic Press)

2. Belmaker, R.H. and Ebstein, R.P. (1979). Adenylate cyclase and the mechanism of lithium action. In: Saletu, B., Berner, P. and Hollister, L. (eds.). Neuropsychopharmacology, pp. 173-184. (London: Pergamon Press)

3. Zohar, J., Ebstein, R.P. and Belmaker, R.H. (1982). Adenylate cyclase as the therapeutic target site of lithium. In: Emrich, H.M., Aldenhoff, J.B. and Lux, H.D. (eds.). Basic Mechanisms in the Action of Lithium. pp. 154-166 (Amsterdam: Excerpta Medica)

4. Bunney, W.E.Jr., Post, R.M., Andersen, K. and Kopanda, R. T. (1977). A neuronal receptor sensitivity mechanism in affective illness: a review of evidence, Commun. Psychopharmacol., 1, 393-405

5. Klawans, H.L. and Rubovits, R.R. (1975), The pharmacology of tardive dyskinesia and some animal models, In: Bassier, J.R., Hippius, H. and Pichot, P. (eds), Proceedings of the IX Congress of CINP. pp, 58-67 (Amsterdam: Excerpta Medica)

6. Klawans, H.L., Weiner, W.S. and Nausieda, P.A. (1977). The effect of lithium on an animal model of tardive dyskinesia. Prog.Neuropsychopharmacol., 1, 53-60

7. Pert, A., Rosenblatt, J.E., Sivit, C., Pert, C.B. and Bunney, W.E. Jr. (1978). Long-term treatment with lithium prevents the development of dopamine receptor supersensitivity. Science, 201, 171-173

8. Gallager, D.W., Pert, A. and Bunney, W.E.Jr. (1978). Haloperidol-induced presynaptic dopamine supersensitivity is blocked by chronic lithium. Nature, 273, 309-312

9. Rosenblatt, J.E., Pert, A., Layton, B. and Bunney, W.E. Jr. (1980). Chronic lithium reduces {^{3}H} spiroperidol binding in rat striatum. Europ.J.Pharmacol., 67, 321-322

10. Bunney, W E.Jr. and Garland, B.L. (1983). Possible receptor

effects of chronic lithium administration. Neuropharmacology, 22, 367-372

11. Staunton, D.A., Magistretti, P.J., Shoemaker, W.J. and Bloom, F.E. (1982). Effects of chronic lithium treatment on dopamine receptors in the rat corpus striatum. I. Locomotor activity and behavioral super-sensitivity. Brain Res., 232, 391-400

12. Seeger, T.F., Gardner, E.L, and Bridger, W.F. (1981). Increase in mesolimbic electrical self-stimulation after chronic haloperidol: reversal by L-Dopa or lithium. Brain Res., 215, 404-409

13. Meller, E. and Friedman, E. (1981). Lithium dissociates haloperidol-induced behavioral supersensitivity from reduced dopac increase in rat striatum. Europ.J.Pharmacol., 76, 25-29

14. Gardner, E.L., Hirschorn, I., Seeger, T.F., Weiss, M. and Makman, M.H. (1980). Comparative effects of lithium on drug-induced supersensitivity. Soc.Neurosc.Abstr., 6, 546

15. Friedman, E., Dallob, A. and Levine, G. (1979). The effect of long-term lithium treatment on reserpine-induced supersensitivity in dopaminergic and serotonergic transmission. Life Sci., 25, 1263-1266

16. Verimer, T., Arnerië, S.P., Long, J.P., Walsh, B.J, and Abou Zeit-Har, M.S. (1981). Effects of ovariectomy, castration, and chronic lithium chloride treatment on stereotyped behavior in rats. Psychopharmacology, 75, 273-276

17. Bowers, M.B.Jr. and Rozitis, A. (1982). Dopamine metabolites and catalepsy after lithium and haloperidol. Europ.J.Pharmacol., 78, 113-115

18. Staunton, D.A., Magistretti, P.J., Shoemaker, W.J., Deyo, S.N. and Bloom, F.E. Effects of chronic lithium treatment on dopamine receptors in the rat corpus striatum. II. No effect on denervation or neuroleptic-induced supersensitivity. Brain Res., 232, 401-412,(1982).

19. Bloom, F.E., Baetge, G., Deyo, S., Ettenberg, A., Koda, L., Magistretti, P.J., Shoemaker, W.J. and Staunton, D.A. (1983). Chemical and physiological aspects of the actions

of lithium and antidepressant drugs. Neuropharmacology, 22, 359-365

20. Reches, A., Wagner, H.R., Jackson, V. and Fahn, S. (1982). Chronic lithium administration has no effect on haloperidol-induced supersensitivity of pre- and post-synaptic dopamine receptors in rat brain. Brain Res., 246, 172-177

21. Wajda, I.J., Banay-Schwartz, M., Manigault, I. and Lajtha A. (1981). Effect of lithium and sodium ions on opiate- and dopamine-receptor binding. Neurochem.Res., 6, 321-331

22. Kafka, M.S., Wirz-Justice, A., Naber, D., Marangos, P. J., O'Donohue, T.L. and Wehr, T.A. (1982). Effect of lithium on circadian neurotransmitter receptor rhythms. Neuropsychobiology, 8, 41-50

23. Tufik, S., Lindsey, C.J. and Carlini, E.A. (1978). Does REM sleep deprivation induce a supersensitivity of dopaminergic receptors in the rat brain? Pharmacology, 16, 98-105

24. Tufik, S. (1981). Increased responsiveness to apomorphine after REM sleep deprivation: supersensitivity of dopamine receptors or increase in dopamine turnover? J.Pharm.Pharmacol., 33, 732-733

25. Mendelson, W.B. et al (1974).The flower pot technique of rapid eye movement (REM) sleep deprivation, Pharmacol. Biochem.Behav., 2, 553-556

26. Tufik, S. (1981). Changes of response to dopaminergic drugs in rats submitted to REM-sleep deprivation. Psychopharmacology, 72, 257-260

27. Rotrosen, J., Angrist, B.M., Wallach, M.B., and Gershon, S. (1972). Absence of serotonergic influence on apomorphine-induced stereotypy. Europ.J.Pharmacol., 20, 133-135

28. Ebstein, R.P., Eliashar, S., Belmaker, R.H., Ben-Uriah, Y. and Yehuda, S. (1980). Chronic lithium treatment and dopamine-mediated behavior. Biol.Psychiatry, 15, 459-467

29. Silva, C.C., Campos, F. and Carlini, E.A. (1980). Aggressive behavior induced by apomorphine in rats

submitted to four stressful situations, Res,Comm,Psychol, Psych,Behav, 5, 353-367

30.   Pert, A. and Bunney, W,E,Jr, (1982). Chronic lithium modulates neurotransmitter receptor sensitivity. In: Emrich, H.M., Aldenhoff, J,B, and Lux, H,D, (eds), Basic Mechanisms in the Action of Lithium. pp. 121-132 (Amsterdam: Excerpta Medica)

31.   Le Douarin, C., Oblin, A., Fage, D. and Scatton, B. (1983). Influence of lithium on biochemical manifestations of striatal dopamine target cell supersensitivity induced by prolonged haloperidol treatment. Europ.J.Pharmacol., 93, 55-62

32.   Belmaker, R.H., Zohar, J, and Levy, A. (1982). Unidirectionality of lithium stabilization on adrenergic and cholinergic receptors. In: Emrich, H.M., Aldenhoff, J. B. and Lux, H.D, (eds). Basic Mechanisms in the Action of Lithium. pp. 146-153. (Amsterdam: Excerpta Medica)

33.   Rosenblatt, J.E., Pert, C.B., Tallman, J.F., Pert, A. and Bunney, W.E.Jr. (1979), The effect of imipramine and lithium on α- and β-receptor binding in rat brain. Brain Res., 160, 186-191

34.   Birmaher, B., Lerer, B. and Belmaker, R.H. (1982). Lithium does not prevent ECS-induced decreases in β-adrenergic receptors. Psychopharmacology, 78, 190-191

Part III
Clinical Aspects
of Long-term
Lithium Treatment

7
Critical issues in the evaluation of long-term lithium treatment

C. L. CAZZULLO AND E. SACCHETTI

INTRODUCTION

How to obtain early assessment of the probability that an individual will benefit from prophylactic treatment with lithium salts critically affects both the clinical and the research fields at three levels of decisions.

First, we become more and more aware that long term lithium treatment implies risks of toxicity and psychological problems which unfavourably influence the patient and his family. Therefore, lithium should be used only when there are no definite somatic and psychologic counter-indications and only for those patients who will probably benefit from the treatment.

Second, other mood-stabilizing therapies that are alternatives to lithium, or that potentiate it are available today (1). Therefore, first choice candidates for such therapies must be selected as rapidly as possible, and should be patients who would not be expected to be lithium responders.

Third, most research into the factors that affect lithium response is based upon comparing patients with different

95

lithium prognoses, and the ability to correctly classify responders and non-responders is a necessary pre-requisite. Therefore, prediction of lithium outcome is one of the major daily decisions to be made. So far, the methodological problems for this have not been surveyed in a way which is completely satisfactory.

Before we can draw any conclusion about whether to continue using lithium or to abandon it, we need to collect evidence that over a period of observation long enough to permit generalization, the patients are indeed lithium non-responders and that the lithium dose was adequate. However, while substantial efforts have been made to carefully define outcome criteria for dividing responders from non-responders, the time- and dose-dependent aspects of this variables have been apparently underestimated. In this paper we report our recent and current studies specifically aimed at better defining the effects of both these variables, time and dose.

1. THE ISSUE OF THE LENGTH OF THE FOLLOW UP

Patients selected for long term lithium treatment suffer from a disease which is by definition recurrent, and therefore have free intervals of variable lengths. The duration of observation is obviously crucial, not only in order to properly select those patients who need lithium prophylaxis because their spontaneous relapse rates are severe enough to require lithium stabilization, but also in order to understand whether or not lithium works.

Follow-up studies of the natural course of the illness (2, 3) seem to be able to individuate patients with high probability of recurrence in the following years and to fix useful time-related criteria for both choosing the lithium candidates and establishing the efficacy of the treatment. Nevertheless, research into long term lithium prophylaxis often underestimates the fact that the length of the follow-up influences the results substantially. Studies about lithium prophylaxis sometimes refer to one and sometimes to several years of treatment, but these differences are generally not taken into account. Thus, in these studies the incidence of lithium responders may be more or less inflated, since patients who simply did not have time enough to relapse are presumed to be lithium responders.   In the same way,   in studies about predictors, some real associations may be overshadowed or some accidental findings may be overemphasized. The three subsequent types of study, which have performed in recent years to test the usefulness of the lithium ratio, are good examples of our thesis.

When we included only the true low-ratio patients - i.e. the individuals with lithium ratio values lower than 0.425 - and the true high lithium ratio patients - i.e. patients with lithium ratio values higher than 0.525-, it appeared that:

1. in the first study (4), with a one-year follow-up, we found only three lithium non-responders, among whom two had low lithium values and one had an intermediate value.

2. in the second study (5), including only patients with two-to-four year follow-ups, almost 90% of non-responders were low lithium rate patients.

3. in the third study (6), including only patients with four-to-six year follow-ups, 25% of high lithium ratio patients had multiple depressive breakdowns.

The specificity (25%, 87.5% & 75%) and the sensitivity

(100%, 90% & 75%) of low lithium ratios for predicting poor lithium outcome in these three studies, that differed in the lengths of follow-up, clearly show (Table 1) to what extent our conclusions may be affected by this chronological variable. In fact it can be seen very clearly that a low lithium ratio as a predictor of poor lithium outcome is quite weak in the first protocol and is too strong and possibly overestimated in the second one, while only in the third protocol was there substantial compensation. Therefore, the lithium ratio may be an important but is not a conclusive factor for lithium outcome.

Table 1.Low lithium ratio as a predictor of poor lithium
        response: influence of the length of the follow-up

STUDY	SPECIFICITY (%)	SENSITIVITY (%)	CORRECT PREDICTION (%)
Cazzullo et al, 1975. (4)	25	100	66.7
Sacchetti et al, 1977. (5)	87.5	90	88.9
Cazzullo et al, 1980. (6)	75	75	75

In order to see what length of follow-up is required to discriminate between responders and non-responders with the reliability which is necessary to consistently reduce classification mistakes, we analyzed a group of patients who were seen each month for five years at the Psycho-biological Branch of the Institute of Clinical Psychiatry of Milan Medical School, and received continuous lithium treatment.

The data collected during that follow-up period permitted us to conclude (6) that 20 to 24 months from the beginning of the lithium therapy are enough to discriminate lithium responders and non-responders with sufficient accuracy, since a substantial number of patients who were classified at those times as non-responders subsequently had multiple affective breakdowns, while only a small number of responders after two years had subsequent, usually isolated, relapses. In fact, the transverse evaluation of lithium response every four months (starting from the end of the first year of prophylaxis) showed an increase in relapsed patients within the first twentyfour months of follow-up (21%, 23%, 31%, 32%, respectively after 12 months and at each of the other time-points up to 2 years). Thereafter the curve for the new relapsers showed a tendency to plateau, meaning that most patients classified as lithium responders after two years on lithium prophylaxis were also protected against affective recurrences during the rest of the follow-up period. Over 74% of the patients classified as lithium non-responders during the first two years had further relapses during the subsequent period of lithium treatment, thus showing that the original classification of 24 months as non-responders was correct.

Comparative analyses of the specificity and sensitivity of the classifications as lithium responders and lithium non-responders at different times, as predictive criteria for subsequent good or poor responses (Table 2), once more show that the patients' classifications after two years of lithium prophylaxis were not only more satisfactory than those based on a shorter period of observation, but also as effective as those based on a longer follow up.

Table 2. Initial good response to lithium as a predictor of
         the subsequent two years lithium outcome:
         influence of the length of the observation time.

FOLLOW UP	SPECIFICITY (%)	SENSITIVITY (%)	CORRECT PREDICTION (%)
12 months	61	66,4	61,7
24 months	67,7	75	70,2
36 months	66,6	80	72,3

In fact the index "responders at twelve months" gave a
correct future lithium prognosis for 61.7% of cases, with
a specificity of 61% and a sensitivity of 66.4%, misclassifications being for the most part due to false positives,
i.e. patients defined as lithium responders but who subsequently had poor responses. Better results were achieved
with a two-year follow-up: the index "responders at two
years" showed, in fact, a substantial improvement in the
incidence of correct classification (70.2%); this gain
was chiefly due to an increase in the specificity (67.7%)
and the sensitivity (75%) of the selection procedure.
Further extention of the follow-up to three years did
not increase correct selection (72.3%): the rise in sensit
ivity (80%) was in fact counteracted by a lower specificity (66.6%) so that the number of correct predictions
of future lithium outcome was equal to the number obtained after two years of lithium treatment.

THE ISSUE OF THE ADEQUACY OF THE LITHIUM REGIMEN

There is now general agreement (7) that the optimal therapeutic plasma lithium levels for patients on long-term lithium treatment are 0.5/0.6 to 1/1.2 mM/l 12 hours after the last dose. This range is usually the reference point for evaluating lithium efficacy. Nevertheless, we think that this measure alone may be not enough and that the intra- to extracellular lithium ratio value for any given patient should be added to this to better individualize the dose regimen. Increased interest in the various in vivo and in vitro indices of the lithium transport processes followed the initial demonstration (8) that intraerythrocyte lithium accumulation correlates better than plasma lithium levels with the concentration of the ion within the CNS, and that the RBC and the neuronal membrane carrier system are quite similar.

After a decade of studies it can be stated that few experimental fields have been so extensively investigated (6, 9, 10, 11, 12, 13). Nevertheless, the studies were involved for the most part with theories of possible pathogenic importance, rather than with possible clinical applications. Paradigmatic examples of this research trend were studies aimed at testing the usefulness of the lithium ratio as a predictor of lithium outcome. Many reports followed our initial observation (4) that the lithium ratio could influence long term lithium treatment in the same way that it was shown to do for antidepressive treatment (14): some results said the lithium ratio was relevant, others said it was not relevant. The studies were more or less aimed at demonstrating that the lithium ratio could or could not express disordered neuronal membrane function of possible pathogenic significance, at least in a definite subgroup of patients.

More attention should be paid to a narrower pharmacokinetic theory, which simply extends to patients the findings in animals that brain lithium concentrations are
better indicated by the Li ratio and consequently hypothes-
izes that, for the same plasma lithium levels, patients
with low lithium ratios are less effectively protected
against affective relapses than patients with high lithium
ratios, simply because the former have inadequate brain
lithium concentrations.

The bulk of our work (6, 11, 12) aimed to test "the
membrane defect" and the "pharmacokinetic" theories seems
to validate this latter hypothesis. When we applied multivariate analysis (11, 12) to data for in vitro lithium
accumulation by RBC from both healthy and subjects with
major affective disorder (MAD), we found that the values
for the RBC lithium accumulation were quite identical
for the healthy and affected group, with no evidence for
any significant direct or interactive gender effect, no
influence of casual error and no influence of the age,
used as a covariate. Subsequent breakdown of MAD patients
according to the unipolar-bipolar dichotomy did not affect
the results. Furthermore, when we searched for possible
linkages between in vitro RBC lithium accumulation and
HLA antigens (11, 12), we found that over 90% of the
subjects with B35 antigen (an antigen present with normal
frequency in MAD patients) were in the group with high
lithium RBC accumulation.   We have interpreted this to
mean that the presence of this antigen by itself leads
to a greater capacity for concentrating lithium inside
the RBC, even though the lack of an absolute association
suggests either a linkage disequilibrium between B35

antigen and some other antigen directly controlling lithium accumulation, or multiple cooperative effects of se
veral antigens of the B locus, each with different quantitative roles in lithium transport. In agreement with
this last hypothesis, lithium accumulation in the RBC
in pairs of healthy siblings who have two, one or no HLA
haplotypes in common, showed that, regardless of which
antigens were present, there were intrapair differences
in accumulation that were greater for the pairs without
any haplotypes in common than for the pairs with two
haplotypes in common.

On the other hand our data would satisfactorily fit a
pharmacokinetic hypothesis. The lithium ratios, measured
in vivo in the MAD population on long term lithium treatment for 4/6 years (6, 12), fall along a normal distribution curve and poor responders occurred with different
frequency in the different lithium ratio classes: patients
with values to the left of the median had a higher frequen
cy of affective breakdowns during lithium prophylaxis
than patients with high lithium ratios, though some non-
responders were found in this last group, too.

This would indicate that high intracellular lithium concentrations, as predicted by the pharmacokinetic postulate,
simply play a facilitating role not a causative one in
adequate stabilization against relapses during lithium
treatment. Clinical progress on lithium, therefore, can
be considered as the resultant of interactions between
adequate lithium concentrations at the sites of action
and specific proclivities of these structures to be positively influenced by the drug.

T he therapeutic implications of this explanation are
obvious. Within a similar context, the significance of

poor lithium outcome appears to potentially differ according to the individual values of the lithium ratios of the patients: non-responders with high lithium ratio levels are the "true" non-responders and at least a sub-group of non-responders with low lithium ratio values are "false" non-responders. Therefore, the management of these two groups of lithium non-responders requires different clinical strategies: if the non-responders have high lithium ratios, alternative or supplementary stabilizing treatment, such as carbamazepine, dipropylacetamide or rubidium salts should be given. If they are unipolar, then typical or atypical antidepressants would be immediately preferred. If the non-responders have low lithium ratios, then high lithium dose regimens might be of therapeutic value.

Future controlled protocols specifically directed at deciding whether or not different lithium ratios require different therapeutic strategies are needed before we can draw any conclusions. Nevertheless our opinion, which is based so far only upon our daily clinical practice, and therefore has to be considered cautiously, is that we can more satisfactorily counteract affective recurrence in lithium non-responders when our therapeutic decisions also take into account the dichotomy "non-responders with high lithium ratios" vs "non-responders with low lithium ratios".

For this point of view, the following three examples are paradigmatic. The first (Figure 1) refers to a unipolar patient with low lithium ratio values: during the first months the patient was maintained without substantial improvement at plasma lithium levels of less than 0.8 mM/l, but always above 0.5 mM/l, which seems to be the

minimum effective plasma levels required for long term
lithium treatment. A subsequent increase in the lithium
dose regimen, to obtain nearly 1 mM/l plasma lithium level
led to satisfactory stabilization. It seems evident that
this patient was a false lithium non-responder, because
the poor outcome during the first part of lithium maintenance was due to the fact that the patient, being a low
lithium ratio patient, had an increased threshold for
the lowest effective dose of lithium.

The second example (Figure 2) is a bipolar patient with
a low lithium ratio. In this case, lithium alone proved
to be thoroughly ineffective when the patient was maintain
ed near either the lower or the higher boundary of the
therapeutic range. Supplementary treatment with carbamazepine initially and then with dipropylacetamide gave
full stabilization, even though the plasma lithium levels
remained close to 0.6 mM/l. In this case it is obvious
that the patient must be classified as a "true non-
responder" and therefore attempts to bypass the pharmacokinetic limitations of the low lithium ratio were un-
successfull, while alternative treatments proved to be
effective.

The third example (Figure 3) had a poor lithium outcome
in spite of a high lithium ratio: the patient, a bipolar
II, during the first months on lithium treatment often
shifted from mild/severe depression to hypomania, whatever the lithium regimen used from time to time. Additional administration of dipropylacetamide seems to have produced beneficial effects, since in the last year of follow-
up only mild mood swings were observed. Our interpretation
of this case was that since the patient had a high lithium
ratio, and was therefore a true lithium non-responder,

he did not improve with increased lithium dosage, whereas the condition of true non-responder obviously did not affect the efficacy of an alternative treatment.

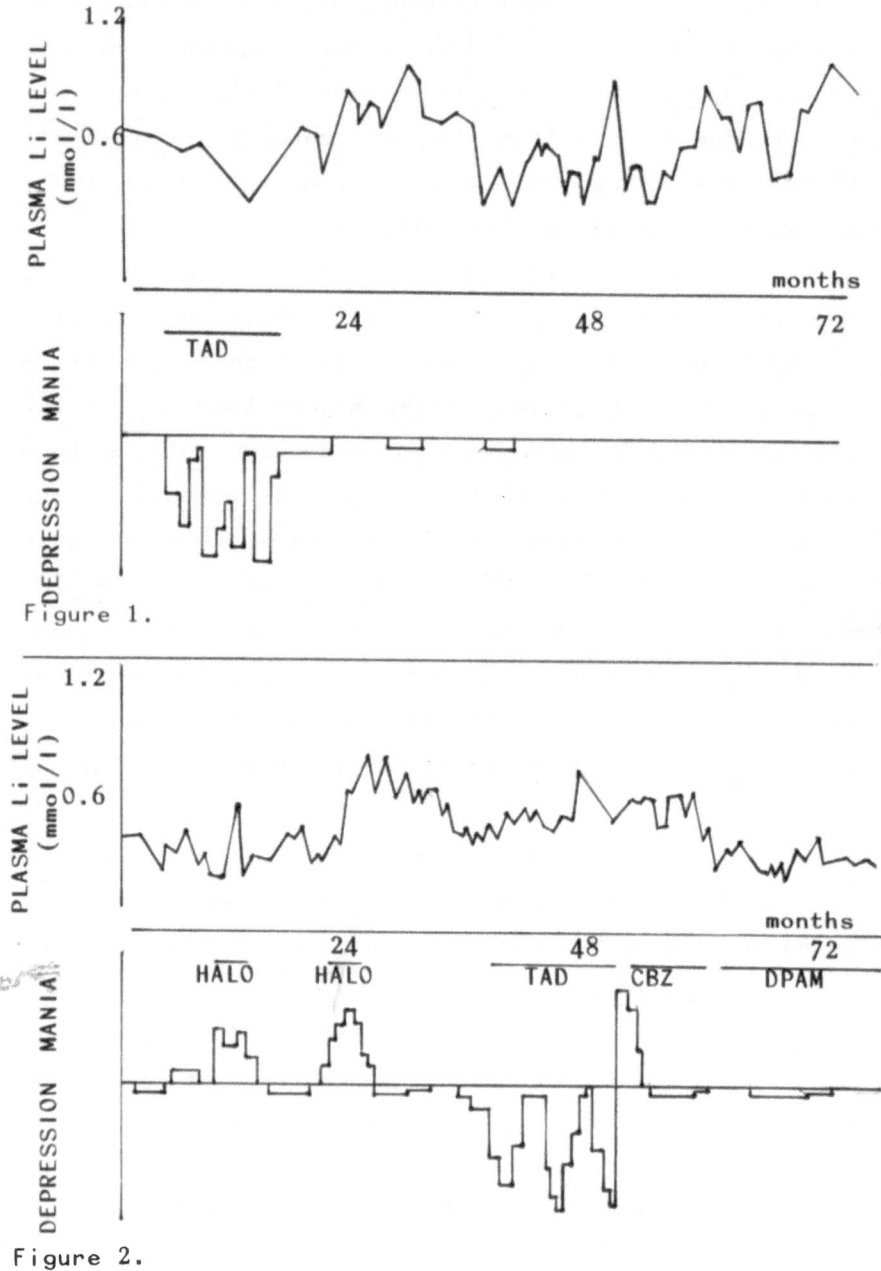

Figure 1.

Figure 2.

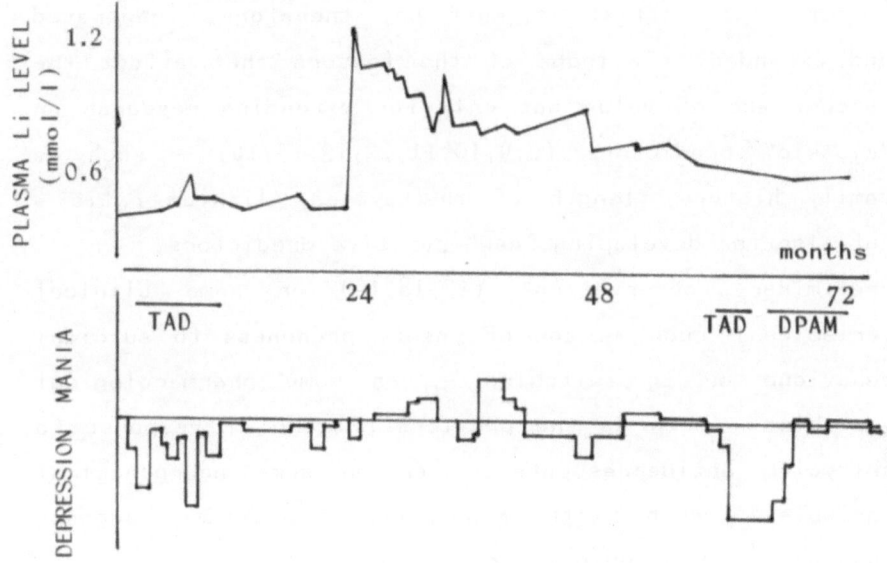

CONCLUSIONS

The evidence presented emphasizes the need for valid operational criteria for properly defining the outcome during
long term lithium treatment and describes an attempt to
improve the reliability of the procedures commonly utilized for this purpose.

Precise codification of the individual's response to lithium prophylaxis is a fundamental prerequisite not only
for any clinical decision centered on lithium but also
for any research attempt to individuate specific features
that might discriminate differences in lithium prognosis.
The need for predictors of lithium response is evermore
an absolute requirement since the extensive use of lithium
salts has revealed that prophylaxis not only shorten the
time spent in illness but also substantially ameliorates
the quality of the life of the patient and his family.

Works to evaluate lithium outcome and to recognize the factors that affect it must be, therefore, integrated and expanded. Knowledge of the factors that affect the outcome are of value not only for extending research on "classic" predictors (6,9,10,11,12,13,15,16) - such as family history, length of the cycles, lithium ratio - but also for developing "new" putative predictors.

Preliminary observations (17,18,19) on some clinical variables - such as age of onset, proneness to suicidal behaviour or to switching -, on some pharmacological variables - such as the previous pattern of response to tricyclic antidepressants -, or on some neurochemical variables - such as the monoaminergic profile - suggest that these areas could be rewarding.

REFERENCES

1. Emrich, H.M. (1982). Prophylactic therapies in affective disorders: mode of action from a clinical point of view. In: Emrich, H.M., Aldenhoff, J.B. and Lux, H.D. (eds). Basic Mechanisms in the Action of Lithium. pp. 202-14. (Amsterdam: Excerpta Medica)

2. Angst, J. and Grof, P.(1979). Selection of patients with recurrent affective illness for a long term study: testing research criteria on prospective follow-up data. In: Cooper, T.B., Gershon, S., Kline, N.S. and Schou, M. (eds). Lithium: Controversies and Unresolved Issues . pp. 355-69. (Amsterdam: Excerpta Medica)

3. Grof, P., Angst, J., Karasek, M. and Keitner, G. (1979). Selection of an individual patient for long term lithium treatment in clinical practice. In: Cooper, T.B., Gershon, S., Kline, N.S. and Schou, M. (eds). Lithium: Controversies and Unresolved Issues. pp. 370-80. (Amsterdam: Excerpta Medica)

4. Cazzullo, C.L., Smeraldi, E., Sacchetti, E. and Bottinelli, S. (1975). Intracellular lithium concentration and clinical response. Brit. J. Psychiat., 126, 298-300.

5. Sacchetti, E., Bottinelli, S., Bellodi, L. et al. (1977). Erythrocyte/plasma lithium ratios. Lancet, i, 908.

6. Cazzullo, C.L., Sacchetti, E. and Smeraldi, E. (1980). New trends on long term lithium treatment in affective disorders. In: Cazzullo, C.L. and Invernizzi, G. (eds). Prevention in Psychiatry. Vol. 1. pp. 115-130. (Milano: Edi Ermes)

7. Amdisen, A. (1979). The standardized twelve-hour serum or plasma concentration in lithium therapy and the use of lithium concentration in lithium intoxication. In: Cooper, T.B., Gershon, S., Kline, N.S. and Schou, M. (eds). Lithium: Controversies and Unresolved Issues. pp. 304-332. (Amsterdam: Excerpta Medica)

8. Frazer, A., Mendels, J., Secunda, S.K. et al.(1973) The prediction of brain lithium concentrations from plasma or erythrocyte measure. J. Psychiat. Res., 10, 1-8.

Carrol, B.J. (1979). Prediction of tretment outcome with lithium. In: Cooper, T.B., Gershon, S., Kline, N.S. and Schou, M. (eds). Lithium: Controversies and Unresolved Issues. pp. 171-97. (Amsterdam: Excerpta Medica)

10. Frazer, A., Mendels, J., Ramsky, T.A. et al. (1979) Erythrocyte concentrations of the lithium ion. In: Cooper, T.B., Gershon, S., Kline, N.S. and Schou, M. (eds). Lithium: Controversies and Unresolved Issues. pp. 198-208. (Amsterdam: Excerpta Medica)

11. Cazzullo, C.L., Bellodi, L., Bonara, P. et al. (1980). Lithium intraerythrocyte accumulation and HLA system. In: Brambilla, F., Racagni, G. and de Wied, D. (eds). Progress in Psychoneuroendocrinology. pp. 487-98. (Amsterdam: Elsevier/North Holland Biomedical Press)

12. Sacchetti, E., Bellodi, L., Catalano, M. and Gu Niu Fan (1981). RBC lithium accumulation and primary affective disorders: clinical and pharmacological considerations. In: Perris, C., Struwe, G. and Jansson, B. (eds). Biological Psychiatry 1981. pp. 1162-6. (Amsterdam: Elsevier/North Holland Biomedical Press)

13. Smeraldi, E., Sacchetti, E. and Bellodi, L. (1980). Uso clinico e modalità di azione dei sali di litio nei disordini affettivi. In: Smeraldi, E. and Sacchetti, E. (eds). La Depressione come Problema Psicobiologico. pp. 185-201. (Milano: Edi Ermes)

14. Mendels, J. and Frazer, A. (1973). Intracellular lithium concentration and clinical response - toward a membrane theory of depression. J. Psychiat. Res., 10, 9-18.

15. Morabito, A., Gasperini, M., Macciardi, F. et al. (1982). Possible relationship between outcome in primary affective disorders treated with lithium and family history. In: Costa, E. and Racagni, G. (eds). Typical

and Atypical Antidepressants: Clinical Practice. pp. 157-
163. (New York: Raven Press)

    16. Mendlewicz, J. (1979). Prediction of treatment
outcome: family and twin studies in lithium prophylaxis
and the question of lithium red blood cell/plasma ratio.
In: Cooper, T.B., Gershon, S., Kline, N.S. and Schou,
M. (eds). Lithium: Controversies and Unresolved Issues.
pp. 226-40. (Amsterdam: Excerpta Medica)

    17. Sacchetti, E., Faravelli, C., Conte, G. et al.
Monoaminergic profiles in major affective disorders and
clinical response to long term lithium treatment. A four-
to-six years follow-up. Submitted for publication.

    18. Sacchetti, E., Vita, A., Conte, G. and Pennati,
A. Lithium prophylaxis in major affective disorders: on
the specificity and sensitivity of some "new" predictors
of treatment outcome. This volume.

    19. Conte, G., Vita, A., Alciati, A. et al. Anti-
depressant-induced switch and outcome to lithium prophylax
is in bipolar patients. This volume.

Supported by CNR Contract N° 82.02298.56.

8
A prospective study of long-term lithium treatment. An interim report

L. SMIGAN AND C. PERRIS

A prospective study of patients who undergo long term lithium treatment to prevent relapses of an affective disorder or of other recurrent psychotic conditions assumed to be influenced by lithium has been going on for a few years at the Department of Psychiatry, Umeå University. The project has been mentioned in previous papers (1, 2). Shortly, its main outlines are as follows:

Eligibility for long term lithium treatment is decided by a team comprised of two psychiatrists, one specialist in internal medicine, and the psychiatric nurses in charge of the lithium clinic who meet once weekly. Criteria for eligibility do not differ from those current used by most lithium clinics and include anamnestic data about the previous course of the illness, and about the frequency of relapses - inclusion criteria - and both anamnestic and present data concerning the somatic state with particular regard to renal- and cardiac function (exclusion criteria).

Patients judged as eligible may enter the treatment first when recovered from any current episode of illness, or at least when improved to such a degree to be able to understand the aim of the treatment and what is expected from them. In practice, such a procedure implies that if a patient is admitted to the hospital, for example for a manic episode, he or she can be treated with lithium during the acute phase of illness but the treatment will be suspended when the patient is re-

(*) Supported (in part) by a grant from the Swedish Medical Research
Council (grant no 21X-5244).

covered and first then the decision will be made whether or not the patient will start long term treatment. We adopted this procedure because we had discovered that the indication for long term lithium treatment had been enlarged in our Department to encompass all patients who were treated acutely with lithium independently of the number of previous episodes, or of the length of the interval between them. We also assumed that the future compliance of the patient would improve if the patient had been able to participate in the decision of starting a long term treatment when mentally well rather than just continuing when recovered a treatment that had been used when he or she was severely ill. Also, since we planned a comprehensive longitudinal monitoring of several biological and psychological functions, we wanted to be able to collect initial data when the patient was euthymic so that each patient represented his own control at the later check-ups.

During the about four years which have elapsed since the project was implemented, only a few exceptions to the above mentioned rule have proved to be necessary. These exceptions have applied mainly to patients with recurrent re-acutizations of a schizoaffective disorder not followed by complete recovery, and to a very few cases with severe, rapidily recurrent affective disorders, again with an uncertain recovery in-between the episodes.

Patients judged eligible for treatment are admitted to either of two acute wards in our Department where a number of beds (five) is constantly reserved for this type of patients. Before starting the treatment, the patients go through a comprehensive screening of several biological and psychological functions as shown in Table 1.

If the results of the biological tests do not contraindicate the treatment then the patient starts the medication and remains in the ward until a satisfactory plasma level has been reached and possible unwanted initial reactions have been excluded. Before starting the treatment the patients are consistently rated by means of appropriate subscales of the CPRS (the Comprehensive Psychopathological Rating Scale (3)) and by using both a self-rating and an observer's scale for side effects developed and currently used in our Department. These ratings are then repeated at the scheduled check-ups.

The successive periodic monitoring of plasma levels is made at the out-patient lithium clinic, or occasionally at other out-patient units

at the periphery of our catchment area. When four months of treatment
have elapsed, the patient is re-admitted to the ward for a check-up
of all the functions which had been examined before starting the treatment. Successive check-ups occur later on at one year of treatment and
afterwards once yearly. If the mental condition of a patient impairs despite the lithium treatment, additional medication can be prescribed by
the team at the lithium clinic. If a patient has to be admitted because
of a more severe relapse, lithium treatment is continued through the
episode of illness independently of which kind of therapy the patient
receives during the phase of relapse.

Table 1. Examination schedule for lithium patients

Psychiatric interview
Somatic examination
Psychopathological rating (CPRS)
Rating by side-effects rating scale
Psychological examinations:
  Memory testing (Cronholm-Molander test)
  Personality inventory (KSP)
Laboratory tests:
  Electrolytes in serum (sodium, potassium, calcium, magnesium).
  Blood analyses (WBC, RBC, platelet count)
  Thyroid function tests (T3, T3-test, TSH, thyroid antibodies)
  Renal function tests (creatinine in serum, creatinine clearance,
                        urine osmolality, DDAVP-test)
  Cortisol in plasma
  ADH in plasma
  ECG
  EEG

In planning this conduct of treatment for our patients there were several expectations:
    a. First of all we expected, as mentioned above, that the fact that
a patient would start the treatment in an euthymic period and when in
a condition to understand the possible advantages of the medication
and the rules bound to it would enhance the motivation to comply pro-

perly with the instructions.

b.   Secondly, we expected that the fact that the patient would participate in a careful monitoring of several biological and psychological
functions would be experienced as a guarantee that we would be able to
promptly detect the possible occurrence of unwanted side-effects and
intervene if necessary. In this respect, it should be mentioned that
the general population in Sweden is well informed about effects and
side-effects of drug treatment in psychiatry through the media that has
given a large space to educational programmes and to debate on such
matter, and that a somewhat negative attitude against prolonged drug
treatment is prevailing.

c.   Thirdly, we are aware that a severe shortcoming of most information concerning the potential occurrence of various side-effects in the
course of lithium treatment consists of the lack of comprehensive initial data. By using the prospective approach, we expect to be able to
add a more accurate information about a time dimension as concerns the
effects of lithium on functions which can be negatively influenced by
the treatment.

So far, fifty-three patients have passed through the one year check-
up after starting the treatment. In the rest of the present article we
will highlight the results obtained in this series as concerns some of
the functions taken into account. More detailed reports concerning the
same series have been published elsewhere (4, 5, 6, 7, 8).

THE SERIES
The series we are referring to is comprised of 20 males and 33 females
in the age range 23-74 years. From a diagnostic point of view, the series is comprised of 16 unipolar and 19 bipolar patients defined according to the criteria given by Perris (9, 10). Eight patients have a diagnosis of cycloid psychosis (11, 12), four patients have a diagnosis of
schizo-affective psychosis according to the criteria by Brockington and
Leff (13) and six patients suffered from recurrent depressive episodes
NUD, that is, patients who did not fulfil the criteria for inclusion in
any of the above mentioned diagnostic subgroups. All the patients in
the series have a long history of recurrent psychotic episodes of an
effective or cycloid nature, or a history of episodes of re-acutization
and of remission of a schizo-affective type without any distinction

whether mostly schizo-manic or schizo-depressive. A few (N=22) of these patients had previously been on long term lithium treatment but a long wash out period had elapsed when they entered the present study. A general survey of the main characteristics of the series is given in Table 2.

Table 2. Patients (N=53)

Diagnosis	N	(%)	M/F	Mean age years	(range)	Previous lithium-treatment	(N)
Unipolar disorder	16	(30)	6/10	51.5	(27 - 74)	8	
Bipolar disorder	19	(36)	8/11	44.0	(25 - 66)	11	
Recurrent depression NUD	6	(11)	1/5	54.0	(40 - 59)	0	
Cycloid psychosis	8	(15)	4/4	41.5	(23 - 61)	5	
Schizo-affective psychosis	4	(8)	1/3	47.5	(32 - 55)	1	
Total	53	(100)	20/33	47.5	(23 - 74)	25	

According to the regime of treatment adopted in our Department it is expected that the patients are kept on a lithium plasma level ranging from 0.6 to 0.8 nmol/ml. The brand of lithium consistently used is a slow-release lithium sulphate preparation.

THE VARIABLES
The variables on which we will comment at this juncture are 'cortisol changes', 'changes in thyroid function tests', 'renal functions' and 'memory functions'. Detailed aspects of methodology are described in the papers mentioned earlier in this article and will not be repeated here. We want to mention, however, that the clinical ratings are made consistently by the same rater (LS), and that the reliability of the other psychological measures has been assessed in previous occasions. As concerns the memory-test battery used by us, it should be mentioned that each subscale is available in two parallel forms. This implies that at least one year has elapsed before the same form is used a second time.

A. Biological measures

a.1. Cortisol changes

The results of several studies have suggested that there is an increase
in plasma cortisol levels in patients suffering from depressive syndromes, and a decrease in cortisol production after recovery (14, 15).
However, only a few studies have taken into account the possible effect
of lithium on the cortisol secretion. Platman and Fieve (16) observed
a significant increase in morning plasma cortisol during the initial
phase of lithium treatment but Sachar et al. (17) did not register significant changes in cortisol levels during short-term lithium treatment.
So far, neither prospective investigations nor studies of long term effects have been reported. The results obtained in our series as concerns this variable are shown in Table 3a, b. It can be seen that whereas the difference among the test occasions is not significant for the
whole group, changes in morning cortisol levels become statistically
significant if the subgroup of patients in which significant changes in
psychopathology did occur is taken into account. Our results suggest
that the decrease of serum cortisol levels observed in our patients is
due to the stabilizing effect of lithium on mood. They also seem to be
in agreement with those of Halmi et al. (18) who suggested that lithium
might blunt the circadian variation of serum cortisol levels by lowering its peak values in the morning.

a.2. Changes in thyroid function tests

The impact of lithium on the thyroid function has been known for a long
time and the occurrence of goitre in patients on long term lithium
treatment has been reported by Schou et al. in 1968 (19). Less frequently hyperthyroidism can also occur as a consequence of lithium treatment
(for a recent review see Smigan et al. (6)). To assess the thyroid function in our patients the following measures have been taken consistently into account: the determination of serum thyroxin, TSH, free thyroxin index, and antithyroid antibodies. In addition, to have a better
estimate of the initial values in our patients a series of healthy controls matched for age and sex have been used for a comparison of the
initial values.

Table 3a. Comparison of CPRS-scores (28 depression items) praelithium
(I), 4 months on lithium (II) and 12 months on lithium (III).
(Wilcoxon matched-pairs signed ranks test).

	$\bar{X} \pm$ SEM		2-tailed p
All patients (N=53)			
CPRS I	15.1 + 1.5		
CPRS II	11.3 $\mp$ 1.3	I vs II	< 0.005
CPRS III	9.4 $\mp$ 1.3	I vs III	< 0.001
All patients except manic/hypomanic (N=48)			
CPRS I	15.9 + 1.5		
CPRS II	11.6 $\mp$ 1.4	I vs II	<0.003
CPRS III	9.7 $\mp$ 1.4	I vs III	<0.001
All depressed patients with CPRS I-III 15% (N=22)			
CPRS I	22.3 + 1.9		
CPRS II	9.9 $\mp$ 1.6	I vs II	< 0.001
CPRS III	6.0 $\mp$ 1.2	I vs III	< 0.001

In the comparison between healthy controls and patients before starting the treatment, TSH was significantly lower (2.55 $\pm$ 1.52 vs 3.39 $\pm$
1.75, p< .02) and the T_3-test significantly higher (1.06 $\pm$ 0.15 vs 0.97
$\pm$ 0.15, p< .01) in the patients than in the healthy controls. The results after four months and one year of lithium treatment in the patient series are shown in Table 4. A significant decrease of S-thyroxin
T_3-test and free thyroxin index occurred after four months of treatment
but the difference between the initial values and those at one year of
treatment was no longer significant. None of the patients in the study
manifested hyperthyroidism. Only one among our patients required treatment with levothyroxine. The results of this part of the study seem to
suggest: first that the incidence of clinical signs of hypothyroidism
is lower than that reported by other authors (about 10% - 20%). Second
that an impairment of the thyroid function occurs very early during
treatment but that a successive improvement can occur later on without
any specific treatment. If these results are confirmed in other prospective studies a practical conclusion would be that levothyroxine
therapy should not be started at the first signs of an impairment of
the thyroid function but should be postponed to later on during the
lithium treatment when thyroid function does not recover spontaneously.

Table 3b. Means (± SEM) of plasma cortisol levels (nmol/l) praelithium
(I), 4 months on lithium (II) and 12 months on lithium (III)
compared by paired t-test.

Cortisol	$\bar{X}$ ± SEM		2-tailed p
All patients except manic/hypomanic (N=48)			
a.m. I	611 ± 28		
a.m. II	561 ± 26	I vs II	n.s.
a.m. III	526 ± 28	I vs III	< 0.05
p.m. I	229 ± 20		
p.m. II	206 ± 18	I vs II	n.s.
p.m. III	210 ± 15	I vs III	n.s.
All depressed patients with CPRS I-III >15% (N=22)			
a.m. I	644 ± 38		
a.m. II	547 ± 37	I vs II	< 0.01
a.m. III	501 ± 41	I vs III	< 0.01
p.m. I	258 ± 32		
p.m. II	218 ± 27	I vs II	n.s.
p.m. III	200 ± 21	I vs III	n.s.
Patients with CPRS I < 10 and CPRS III ≤ 10 (N=12)			
a.m. I	640 ± 60		
a.m. III	615 ± 48		n.s.
p.m. I	193 ± 31		
p.m. III	196 ± 30		n.s.
Patients with CPRS I > 10 and CPRS III ≤ 5 (N=14)			
a.m. I	625 ± 41		
a.m. III	499 ± 38		< 0.005
p.m. I	250 ± 45		
p.m. III	185 ± 24		n.s.

Table 4. Comparison of values of thyroid function tests after 4 and 12
months on lithium with praelithium values by paired t-test.
Mean values ± SD   (N=51)

Time on lithium (months)	Before lithium treatment	4 months on lithium	12 months on lithium
S-thyroxin (mmol/l)	101.1 ± 24.5	93.0 ± 24.5[**]	100.3 ± 24.1
T_3-test (work units)	1.06 ± 0.15	1.01 ± 0.15[*]	1.04 ± 0.26
Free thyroxin index (work units)	106.2 ± 27.5	92.5 ± 23.0[***]	102.1 ± 31.3
S-TSH (mU/l)	2.55 ± 1.52	3.22 ± 2.06	3.03 ± 1.60

[*]$p < 0.05$;   [**]$p < 0.01$;   [***]$p < 0.001$

a.3. Renal functions

The possibility that long term lithium treatment might induce not only
functional changes but also irreversible renal damage has been a matter
of much concern during the last years (for recent rev. (21, 22)). Most of
the information on this subject has been gathered in cross-sectional
studies of patients who had been on lithium treatment for several years
or in comparisons between results obtained in patients on lithium and
in healthy controls. More recent data (23, 24) suggest, however, that
functional changes are mostly small, and of little clinical significance.
In particular, in a four years follow-up of patients who had shown an
impaired concentrating ability while on lithium and who had stopped lithium treatment, Smigan and Perris could show a return to a normal function, also in patients who had shown very low osmolality values. Obviously, these findings do not exclude that single patients might still
risk an irreversible functional impairment and also parenchimal damage,
but this risk has probably been overestimated especially if a strict
conduct of treatment is adhered to and periodical check-ups of the renal function are planned.

The results concerning serum creatinine, creatinine clearance and
maximum urine osmolality obtained in our prospective series are shown
in Table 5.

Table 5. Comparison of means of serum creatinine, creatinine clearance
and maximal concentrating ability (DDAVP-test) by paired t-
test. (N=53).

Variable	Before li treatm (I) $\bar{X}$+SEM	4 months on li (II) $\bar{X}$+SEM	12 months on li (III) $\bar{X}$+SEM	2-tailed p		
Serum creatinine (μg/l)	77.9+1.9	84.3+1.9	82.0+2.0	I vs II	< 0.001	
				I vs III	< 0.05	
				II vs III	n.s.	
Creatinine clea-rance (ml/m2/min)	127.6+5.3	106.0+4.1	113.7+5.5	I vs II	< 0.001	
				I vs III	< 0.05	
				II vs III	n.s.	
Maximum urine osmolality (mmol/kg H_2O)	800.7+20.3	702.0+20.0	732.2+16.9	I vs II	< 0.001	
				I vs III	< 0.001	
				II vs III	n.s.	

In line with the results obtained from other authors a small decrease of both the tubular and the glomerular function has been found, but such am impairment does not seem to progress during the first year of lithium therapy. Multiple regression analyses which have taken into account a possible interfering effect of age, sex, and the occurrence of complementary treatments suggest that these factors do not contribute to the regression.

Table 6. Median values of memory scores before lithium (I) and after 4 months (II) and 12 months (III) respectively. (Wilcoxon matched-pairs signed ranks test)

Test variables	N	Median	Interquartile range		Significance
Immediate memory score					
30 Figure Test I	53	23.8	7.0		
-"- II	53	25.1	6.0	I vs II	n.s.
-"- III	35	25.2	8.0	I vs III	n.s.
30 Word Pair Test I	53	20.0	10.0		
-"- II	53	19.0	7.0	I vs II	n.s.
-"- III	35	17.7	8.0	I vs III	n.s.
30 Person-Data Test I	53	13.2	8.0		
-"- II	53	15.0	7.0	I vs II	< 0.05
-"- III	35	15.1	11.0	I vs III	n.s.
30 Face Test I	48	14.1	9.0		
-"- II	48	16.8	10.0	I vs II	< 0.001
-"- III	34	18.5	9.0	I vs III	< 0.001
Delayed memory score					
30 Figure Test I	53	21.9	8.0		
-"- II	52	22.7	6.0	I vs II	n.s.
-"- III	35	23.2	8.0	I vs III	n.s.
30 Word Pair Test I	53	13.6	10.0		
-"- II	52	12.9	9.0	I vs II	n.s.
-"- III	34	14.7	11.0	I vs III	n.s.
30 Person-Data Test I	53	12.1	9.0		
-"- II	52	13.6	6.0	I vs II	< 0.02
-"- III	35	12.6	10.0	I vs III	n.s.
30 Face Test I	48	12.5	10.0		
-"- II	48	14.5	11.0	I vs II	< 0.05
-"- III	34	15.5	12.0	I vs III	< 0.02

B. Psychological functions

b.1. Memory functions

A still unsettled issue is whether lithium treatment does affect memory functions and if so to what extent. The controversial findings available in the literature have been summarized in a previous occasion and will not be repeated here (23, 4). None of the reports by other authors has been concerned with a prospective investigation, and only in very few of them details about the mental state of the patients at the time of the memory tests are given in a satisfactory way.

Patients in our series have been tested by means of a well established Swedish memory test battery (25) before starting the treatment and later on after four and twelve months of treatment. At each test-occasion the patients have also been rated by means of the CPRS. The results of this part of the study are summarized in Table 6. It can be seen that if anything, lithium treatment has produced a slight but statistically significant improvement in several of the functions explored. A multiple regression analysis in which several variables have been taken into account suggests that a young age and a low initial CPRS score are factors which contribute to the results obtained with the memory test battery.

CONCLUSIONS

The results presented at this junction refer to only one part of a larger prospective study that is going on at our Department. Since the duration of the follow up so far is not longer than one year and since the series is still small, they should be interpreted cautiously.

Our experience as concerns both the variables reported above and the general conduct of treatment adopted in our Department can, provisionally by summarized as follows:

1. In line with expectations, the adoption of a particular structure for conducting long term lithium treatment seems to give a positive result. Patients feel satisfied in getting an opportunity of deciding about their participation in a long term treatment when they no longer are under the pressure of a psychopathological condition. This possibility seems to enhance their motivation and to minimize the risk of non-compliance.

2. None of the variables investigated so far, not only those report-

ed in this article, but also other reported elsewhere (for example ECG
(8)) has shown the occurrence of pathological changes which could be
due to the lithium treatment. The functional impairment of some functions that has emerged in some of our investigations seems to be small
and of little clinical significance.

3. The prospective nature of our study has permitted to evidentiate
that some minor functional changes occur very early in the treatment
but that they do not progress further, at least within the time limits
of our study.

4. A continued follow up of the patients entering our study will probably allow us to be able to elucidate time aspects as concerns the occurrence and development of certain side-effects during lithium treatment.

REFERENCES
1. Perris, C. and Smigan, L. (1980). Lithium and the kidney: our present knowledges and some guidelines for the future. Riv. Psichiat., 15,
11-20.
2. Bucht, G., von Knorring, L., Smigan, L. and Wahlin, A. (1981). Control of lithium treatment - experiences from a lithium clinic. Nord.
psykiat. tidskr., 35, 160-165.
3. Åsberg, M., Perris, C., Schalling, D. and Sedvall, G. (1978). The
CPRS - Development and applications of a psychiatric rating scale. Acta
psychiat. scand., suppl. 271.
4. Smigan, L. and Perris, C. (1983a). Memory functions and prophylactic treatment with lithium. Psychol. Med. 13, 529-536.
5. Smigan, L. and Perris, C. (1983b). Cortisol changes in long-term
lithium therapy. Neuropsychobiology, in press.
6. Smigan, L., Wahlin, A., Jacobsson, L. and von Knorring, L. (1983a).
Lithium therapy and thyroid function tests: a prospective study. Intern.
Pharmacopsychiat., in press.
7. Smigan, L., Bucht, G., von Knorring, L., Perris, C. and Wahlin, A.
(1983b). Long term lithium therapy and renal functions: a prospective
study. Intern. Pharmacopsychiat., in press.
8. Bucht, G., Smigan, L. and Wahlin, A. (1983). ECG-changes during
lithium therapy: a prospective study. Intern. Pharmacopsychiat., in
press.

9. Perris, C. (1966). A study of bipolar and unipolar recurrent depressive psychoses. Acta psychiat. scand., suppl. 194.

10. Perris, C. (1973). The heuristic value of a distinction between
bipolar and unipolar affective disorders. In: Angst, J. (ed). Classification and Prediction of Outcome of Depression. pp. 75-98. (Stuttgart:
Schattauer).

11. Perris, C. (1974). A study of cycloid psychosis. Acta psychiat.
scand., suppl. 253.

12. Brockington, I.F., Perris, C. and Meltzer, H.Y. (1982). Cycloid
psychoses: Diagnosis and heuristic value. J. nerv. ment. Dis., 170,
651-656.

13. Brockington, I.F. and Leff, J. (1979). Schizoaffective psychoses:
Definition and incidence. Psychol. Med., 9, 91-99.

14. Gibbons, J.L. (1964). Cortisol secretion rate in depressive illness. Arch. gen. Psychiat., 10, 572-577.

15. Sachar, E.J. (1978). Neuroendocrine responses to psychotropic
drugs. In: Lipton, M. et al. (eds). Psychopharmacology. A Generation of
Progress. (New York: Raven Press).

16. Platman, R.S. and Fieve, R.R. (1968). Lithium carbonate and plasma cortisol response in the affective disorders. Arch. gen. Psychiat.,
18, 591-594.

17. Sachar, E.J., Hellman, L., Kream, J., Fukushima, D.K. and Gallagher,
T.F. (1970). Effect of lithium carbonate therapy on adrenocortical activity. Arch. gen. Psychiat., 32, 304-307.

18. Halmi, K.A., Noyes, R. and Millard, S.A. (1972). Effect of lithium
on plasma cortisol and adrenal response to adrenocorticotropin in man.
Clin. Pharmacol. Ther., 13, 699-703.

19. Schou, M., Amdisen, A., Jensen, S.E. and Olsen, T. (1968). Occurrence of goitre during lithium treatment. Brit. Med. J., 3, 719-723.

20. Hullin, R.P. (1978). The plasma of lithium in biological psychiatry. In: Johnson, F.N. and Johnson, S. (eds). Lithium in Medical Practice.
pp. 434-454. (Lancaster: MTP Press).

21. Vestergaard, P. and Amdisen, A. (1981). Lithium treatment and kidney function. Acta psychiat. scand., 63, 333-345.

22. Hansen, H.E. (1981). Renal toxicity of lithium. Drugs, 22, 461-476.

23. Smigan, L. and Perris, C. (1982). Some aspects of long term lithium therapy. Read at the XXXV Congr. Ital. Soc. Psychiat., Forte Vil-
lage (Cagliari), Sept. 30-Oct. 2, 1982, in press in the proceedings.

24. Decina, P., Oliver, J.A., Sciacca, R.R., Colt, E. and Fieve, R.R. (1983). Effect of lithium therapy on glomerular filtration rate. Am. J. Psychiat., 140, 1065-1067.

25. Cronholm, B. and Molander, L. (1957). Memory disturbances after electroconvulsive therapy. Acta psychiat. scand., 31, 280-306.

9
Lithium dosage and prophylaxis. A double-blind controlled study

A. COPPEN AND K. WOOD

SUMMARY

In a prospective double-blind trial we examined the affective morbidity and side-effects of 72 patients who were randomly allocated either to continue with their usual dose of lithium or to receive either a 25% or 50% reduction in lithium dosage. Patients who underwent a dosage reduction with consequently lower plasma lithium levels (0.45 - 0.79 mmol/l) had significantly decreased affective morbidity. Total subjective side-effects score and tremor were also reduced. No change in affective morbidity was observed during the trial in patients whose dosage was not altered. These changes were observed in both unipolar and bipolar patients.

It was concluded that a once-a-day dosage with a sustained release lithium preparation that maintained a 12-hour plasma level of about 0.6 mmol/l is both more effective and produces less side effects than does conventional dosages.

INTRODUCTION

Most investigations studying the efficacy of lithium for prophylaxis have been carried out using a dosage regime, once or twice daily, that produces a plasma concentration of between 0.8 and 1.2 mmol/l 12 h after the last dose (1). It is well established that severe side-effects and toxic reactions occur with dosages that produce 12 h plasma lithium concentrations of 1.5 mmol/l or more. The minimum plasma concentration of lithium needed for effective prophylaxis has not been studied in prospective, double-blind investigations although some authors have suggested that the minimum effective dosage may be lower than previously thought and patients may be maintained satisfactorily in some cases with 12 h lithium concentrations as low as 0.4 mmol/l (2).

In view of these findings and the narrow margin between established therapeutic concentrations and toxicity, it was decided that a double-blind prospective investigation should be initiated to study the consequent changes in affective morbidity and side-effects when patients, previously maintained at dosages to give a 12 h plasma lithium concentration of 0.8 - 1.2 mmol/l, had their dosage of lithium reduced by 25% or 50%.

METHODS AND PATIENTS

Design of the Trial

Eighty-eight patients attending our lithium clinic agreed to take part in the trial and these patients were then randomly allocated either to remain on their previous dosage (mean 12 h plasma lithium concentration 0.86 ± 0.2 mmol/l) or to receive approximately a 25% or 50% reduction of lithium. The reduction was approximate as the smallest unit of lithium carbonate (sustained release preparation; Priadel, Delandale Laboratories, Canterbury) was ½ tablet of 200 mg. No patient was allowed to fall below a dosage that would give a 12 h plasma lithium concentration of 0.45 mmol/l. The lithium carbonate was given once daily at night. No patient was adjusted to give an increased dosage. Different amounts of lithium carbonate were packed into identical looking capsules to maintain the double-blind nature of the trial. A research co-ordinator (who was not involved in the clinical assessment of patients) monitored the plasma levels of lithium.

During the trial period of at least one year, most patients were
assessed at 6 - 8 weekly intervals and their affective morbidity and
side-effects were compared with a similar period immediately preceeding
the trial. If the patients were affectively ill they were assessed
at weekly intervals. The patients' affective morbidity over the trial
period was assessed using the affective morbidity index (AMI). This is
a measure related not only to the severity of the episode but also to
the time spent with such an episode. It is therefore based on a frequent
assessment of the patients' clinical state. On each occasion that the
patients attended the clinic, their affective state was plotted on the
Affective Disorders Chart (3) using a 4-point scale as follows :

    0 = No conspicuous depression or mania
    1 = Mild depression or mania
    2 = Moderate depression or mania
    3 = Severe depression or mania

A line was drawn between the points indicating the degree of affective
disorder at each attendance at the clinic. The area under the curve
was then calculated and divided by the relevant time period to give the
AMI.

An approximate guide to the interpretation of AMI is as follows :
an AMI of < 0.2 indicated nil or slight morbidity; an AMI of 0.2 - 0.4
indicates mild morbidity and an AMI of > 0.4 indicated moderate to severe
morbidity during the period of the trial.

The number and severity cf side-effects were assessed using a
check-list (4) that was completed by the patient at each visit to the
clinic. The mean side-effect score was calculated for each patient
during the present investigation both during the trial and for the same
period preceeding the trial.

Patients
These were unipolar or bipolar patients who had suffered 3 or more
episodes of a major affective illness. All patients had been receiving
lithium for a minimum of one year and the majority had been receiving

lithium for many years. The patients were classified for the purpose of analyses, into 4 groups according to their plasma lithium concentration over the trial period :

1. 20 patients with plasma lithium concentration of 0.45 - 0.59 mmol/l (mean : 0.52 + 0.02 mmol/l)

2. 33 patients with plasma lithium concentration of 0.60 - 0.79 mmol/l (mean : 0.70 + 0.01 mmol/l)

3. Groups 1 and 2 combined, that is 53 patients with a plasma lithium concentration = 0.79 mmol/l (mean : 0.63 + 0.02 mmol/l)

4. 19 patients whose dosage was not adjusted, that is with a plasma lithium concentration of = 0.80 mmol/l (mean : 0.92 + 0.02 mmol/l)

RESULTS

Sixteen patients failed to complete the trial : 7 patients were discontinued because of deterioration in their clinical state (all had onset of depressive symptoms). Of these, 3 had plasma lithium levels of between 0.45 and 0.59 mmol/l; 1 between 0.60 and 0.70 and 3 had levels of = 0.80. The other patients discontinued for a variety of reasons, e.g. moving away from the area.

The affective morbidity of the unipolar and bipolar patients before and during the trial are shown in Table 1. The patients with plasma lithium concentrations = 0.79 mmol/l had a significant decrease (34%) in their affective morbidity during the trial period. The patients with plasma concentrations of 0.45 - 0.59 mmol/l also had a mean decrease of 34%; patients with plasma concentrations = 0.80 mmol/l showed little change.

Unipolar patients maintained with plasma levels of $\leq$ 0.79 mmol/l showed a significant decrease in morbidity of 34%. Patients with a plasma level of 0.45 - 0.59 mmol/l had a mean decrease of similar magnitude. Those unipolar patients with a level of $\geq$ 0.80 mmol/l had an increase in morbidity of 17%.

Table 1. Affective morbidity index for all patients before and during
the trial period. Results expressed as mean $\pm$ S.E.M.

Plasma lithium level during trial (mmol/l)	N	Affective morbidity index Pre-trial	During trial	% change
0.45 - 0.59	20	0.14 $\pm$ 0.04	0.09 $\pm$ 0.03	- 33.8
0.60 - 0.79	33	0.26 $\pm$ 0.05	0.18 $\pm$ 0.03	- 33.3
= 0.79	53	0.22 $\pm$ 0.04	0.14* $\pm$ 0.02	- 33.6
= 0.80	19	0.24 $\pm$ 0.06	0.24 $\pm$ 0.05	+ 0.3

*Significant reduction from 'pre-trial' morbidity, p < 0.02

There was a 30% reduction in those bipolar patients with reduced
lithium plasma levels during the trial.

The mean total side-effect scores for both unipolar and bipolar
patients before and during the trial period are shown in Table 2.
Those patients with a plasma lithium concentration of = 0.79 mmol/l
showed a small but significant reduction in side-effects. Items listed
on the side-effects checklist that are particularly related to lithium
treatment were examined and the tremor scores are shown in Table 3.
Patients in the 3 lower lithium concentration groups showed a decrease
of more than 20% in tremor. Those patients with a lithium level of
= 0.80 mmol/l showed a significant increase (37%) in this troublesome
side-effect.

In order to assess whether the beneficial effects of a reduced
lithium plasma level were due to patients receiving additional
psychotropic medication, an analysis was made of the neuroleptics and
antidepressant drugs prescribed during the last 3 months of the trial
and compared with those prescribed in the 3 month period preceeding the
trial. In the patients with a plasma lithium concentration of = 0.79
mmol/l, 4 patients (7.5%) receiving a neuroleptic before the trial were

still taking the drug in the last 3 months of the trial. Eight patients (15%) receiving an antidepressant before the trial and 7 patients (13%) received the drug during the last 3 months of the trial.

Table 2.   Total side-effect score for all patients before and during the trial period. Results expressed as mean $\pm$ S.E.M.

Plasma lithium level during trial (mmol/l)	N	Total side-effects score		% change
		Pre-trial	During trial	
0.45 - 0.59	20	6.6 $\pm$ 1.0	5.8 $\pm$ 1.1	- 11.4
0.60 - 0.79	33	7.6 $\pm$ 1.3	7.0 $\pm$ 1.3	- 7.6
= 0.79	53	7.2 $\pm$ 0.9	6.6[*] $\pm$ 0.9	- 9.0
= 0.80	19	6.7 $\pm$ 1.3	8.0 $\pm$ 1.8	+ 19.2

[*]Significant reduction from 'pre-trial' morbidity, $p < 0.05$

Table 3.   Tremor score for all patients before and during the trial period. Results expressed as mean $\pm$ S.E.M.

Plasma lithium level during trial (mmol/l)	N	Side-effects : Tremor score		% change
		Pre-trial	During trial	
0.45 - 0.59	20	0.51 $\pm$ 0.14	0.40 $\pm$ 0.13	- 21.1
0.60 - 0.79	33	0.54 $\pm$ 0.10	0.40[*] $\pm$ 0.09	- 27.1
= 0.79	53	0.53 $\pm$ 0.08	0.40[**] $\pm$ 0.07	- 25.0
= 0.80	19	0.46 $\pm$ 0.10	0.63[***] $\pm$ 0.15	+ 36.8

[*]Significant reduction from 'pre-trial' score, $p < 0.02$

[**]Significant reduction from 'pre-trial' score, $p < 0.005$

[***] Significant increase from 'pre-trial' score, $p < 0.01$

In the group of patients with a plasma lithium concentration of = 0.80 mmol/l 3 patients (16%) received a neuroleptic before and 2 patients (11%) received a neuroleptic during the last 3 months of the trial period. Four patients (21%) received an antidepressant before the trial and 7 patients (37%) received the drug during the last 3 months of the trial.

DISCUSSION

The results of the present investigation indicate a striking reduction in the affective morbidity of patients who undergo a reduction of their daily lithium dose : it was not due to patients receiving additional psychotropic medication. This effect was apparent even in the patients with the lowest lithium concentration (= 0.59 mmol/l) and was particularly marked in the unipolar patients.

Reduced plasma concentrations of lithium were associated with a decrease in side-effects. The mean total side-effects score of the lithium-treated patients were similar to that of the general population (5). With lower doses (and consequently lower plasma concentrations) the troublesome unwanted effect of tremor was significantly reduced.

It has been reported (6) that a once-a-day regime requires approximately 15% less lithium to be administered than a twice-a-day regime to maintain similar plasma levels. Apart from encouraging compliance, a once rather than a twice-a-day regime significantly reduces the 24 h urinary output (7) and reduces the risk of renal damage (8). A reduction of the once-a-day regime may therefore be of more benefit than the twice-a-day system.

These results suggest that the reduction of lithium dosage should be investigated further since the lowest plasma concentration of lithium studied (not lower than 0.45 mmol/l) in this investigation was generally associated with a low affective morbidity and a low side-effects score. The effectiveness of a plasma lithium concentration within the range of 0.35 - 0.45 mmol/l is worthy of further investigation in a prospective double-blind manner.

In conclusion, lower doses of lithium appear to be beneficial in
increasing the effectiveness of treatment by reducing morbidity and
troublesome side-effects. These results should encourage the prudent use
of one of the most powerful psychotropic drugs and indicate that a
once-a-day dosage giving a 12 h lithium concentration of about o.6
mmol/l is the optimum dosage.

ACKNOWLEDGEMENTS
We are grateful to Drs. Abou-Saleh and Milln; to Mrs. Cynthia Swade and
Mrs. Janet Harwood for measuring the plasma levels of lithium; to
Mr. Bailey for co-ordinating the study; to Mrs. Carlisle and her pharmacy
staff, to Mrs. Rosemary Bishop for carrying out reception dutues in the
Lithium Clinic; to Mrs. Joan Owen for secretarial assistance and to
Mrs. Maryse Metcalfe for valuable advice.

We thank the Medical Research Council for financial support and
Delandale Laboratories for the supplies of Priadel. Lastly, and by no
means least, we thank all the patients who took part in this trial.

REFERENCES
Coppen, A., Noguera, R., Bailey, J., Burns, B.H., Swani, M.S., Hare, E.H.,
Gardner, R. and Maggs, R. (1971). Prophylactic lithium in affective
disorders : controlled trial. Lancet, ii, 275 - 9.

Jerram, T.C. and McDonald, R. (1978). Plasma lithium control with
particular reference to minimum effective levels In : Johnson, F.N.
and Johnson, S. (eds). Lithium in Medical Practice. pp. 407 - 13.
(Lancaster, MTP Press)

Coppen, A., Peet, M., Bailey, J., Noguera, R., Burns, B.H., Swani, M.S.,
Maggs, R. and Gardner, R. (1973). Double-blind and open prospective
studies of lithium prophylaxis in affective disorders. Psychiat. Neurol.
Neurochir., (Amst) 76, 501 - 10.

Ghose, K. (1977). Lithium salts : therapeutic and unwanted effects.
Brit. J. Hosp. Med., 18, 578 - 83.

Abou-Saleh,M. and Coppen, A. (1983). Subjective side-effects of amitritpyline and lithium in the affective disorders. Brit. J. Psychiat., 142, 391 - 97.

Plenge, P., Mellerup, E.T., Bolwig, T.G., Brun, C., Hetmar, O., Ladefoged, J., Larsen, S. and Refaelson, O.J. (1982). Lithium treatment: does the kidney prefer one daily dose instead of two? Acta Psychiat. Scand., 66, 121 - 28.

Perry, P.J., Dunner, F.J., Hahn, R.L., Tsuang, M.T. and Berg, M.J. (1981). Lithium kinetics in single daily dosing. Acta Psychiat. Scand., 64, 281 - 94.

Plenge, P., Mellerup, E.T. and Nørgaard, T. (1981). Functional and structural rat kidney changes caused by peroral or parenteral lithium treatment. Acta Psychiat. Scand., 63, 303 - 13.

10
Lithium discontinuation in bipolar illness: a double-blind prospective controlled study

J. MENDLEWICZ

ABSTRACT

Twenty eight bipolar manic depressive patients who had been treated with lithium carbonate for at least five years without affective relapse took part in a double blind controlled lithium discontinuation study. Patients were randomly allocated to lithium carbonate or placebo (within two weeks to avoid abrupt lithium withdrawal) and followed up to one year in a outpatient clinic. Fictive lithium plasma levels were provided for placebo patients as to maintain blindness of the treating physician. Clinical relapses were recorded for all patients as well as side effects using the Hamilton rating scale, for depression the Bunney-Hamburg scale (for mania) and a lithium side effects questionnaire.

No apparent withdrawal symptoms were noted, but the rate of relapse was significantly greater in the placebo group when compared to the lithium treatment group. These results are discussed with special reference to the patients clinical and social background.

INTRODUCTION

Because of the potential physical and psychological hazards of long term lithium utilisation and the request of many patients on lithium prophylactic treatment to interrupt

such treatment, we have decided to perform a lithium
discontinuation study in bipolar manic depressive patients
after obtaining their informed consent.

SAMPLE AND METHOD

Patients selected in this study were bipolar patients
according to the R.D.C. criteria (1), who had been treated
with lithium carbonate alone for at least five years
without any acute relapses necessitating hospitalisation or
major changes in medication (ie. the addition of
neuroleptics or antidepressants). These patients also
showed only minor side effects from the lithium treatment.
Twenty eight bipolar patients on lithium prophylactic
treatment were thus randomly allocated to placebo (N=14) or
lithium (N=14), the allocation procedure being done over
a two weeks period to avoid any potential acute withdrawal
effects. The study was conducted in a double blind fashion,
fictive lithium plasma levels being provided for the
placebo patients. Patients were followed-up for 12 months
with monthly plasma lithium levels and clinical evaluations
using the Hamilton Rating Scale for depression (2), the
Bunney-Hamburg Scale for mania (3) and a lithium side
effects scale.

RESULTS

Table 1. Recurrence of affective episodes during follow-up
         period of twelve months

	Depression	Mania	Mixed	Total
Placebo Patients N=14	8	3	1	12
Lithium Patients N=14	1		1	2

Table 1 compares the rates of affective relapses. In the
lithium group, only 2 patients had an affective relapse
(1 depression, 1 mixed state) for 12 patients in the

placebo group. The affective relapses in the placebo group
were as follows : 8 patients with depression, 3 patients
with mania and 1 patient with a mixed episode.

Table 2. Clinical characteristics of relapsing patients on
         placebo

Clinical Diagnosis	Years	Sex	Lithium Therapy (months)	Affective Episodes <LI	Relapse Episode	Relapse Interval
Bipolar I	51	F	132	9	Depression	5 days
Bipolar I	47	M	88	6	Mania	17 days
Bipolar I	58	F	141	13	Mania	28 days
Bipolar I	43	F	97	8	Depression	30 days
Bipolar II	49	F	111	5	Depression	31 days
Bipolar II	54	M	77	12	Depression	60 days
Bipolar II	38	F	123	7	Depression	72 days
Bipolar I	42	F	115	8	Mania	95 days
Bipolar II	61	M	98	11	Mixed	156 days
Bipolar I	57	F	142	6	Depression	180 days
Bipolar II	58	M	121	7	Depression	245 days
Bipolar	63	F	93	9	Depression	340 days

The clinical characteristics of placebo relapsing patients
are listed in Table 2. Patients were subdivided in bipolar
I and II. Their age varied from 38 years to 63 years, there
were 8 female patients for 4 males. The patients had been
on lithium prophylactic treatment from 77 months to 142
months and the number of affective episodes before the
initiative of lithium therapy varied from 5 to 13 affective
episodes. These clinical and demographic characteristics of
the placebo, patients were comparable to those of the
patients remaining on lithium treatment. The type of
affective relapse and the relapse interval (time between
complete lithium withdrawal and relapse) are also listed
in Table 2. Eight patients presented a depressive relapse
with a relapse interval ranging from 5 days to 340 days.
Three patients had a manic relapse after 17 days to 95 days

and the patient with a mixed episode relapsed after 156
days.

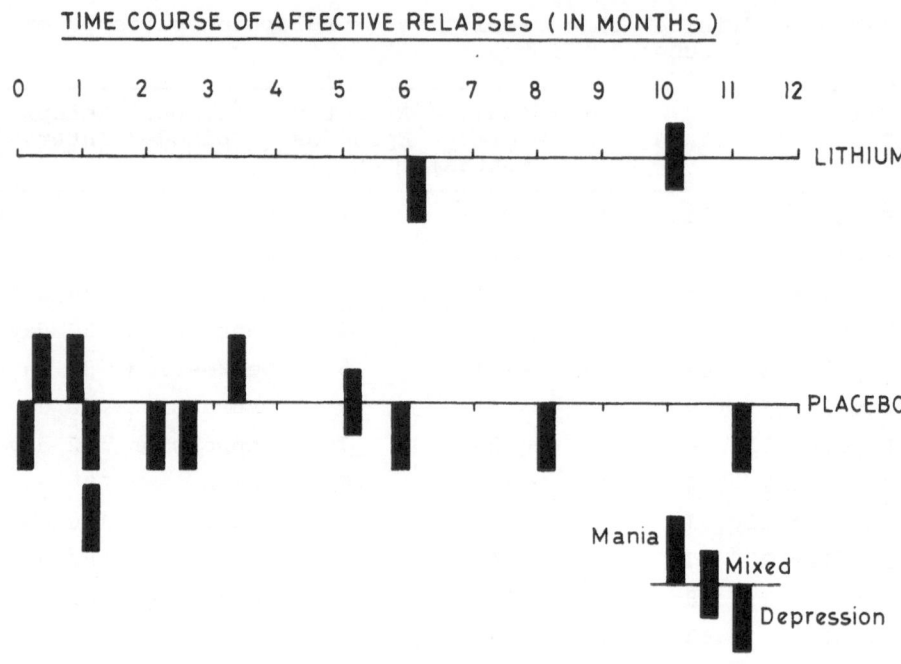

TIME COURSE OF AFFECTIVE RELAPSES (IN MONTHS)

FIGURE 1 illustrates the long term course of affective
         relapses in the lithium and placebo group.

Most affective relapses wether of depressed or manic type
occur precociously before 4 months after lithium
discontinuation while relapses in patients on lithium
treatment appear later, after a 6 months'period of
observation.

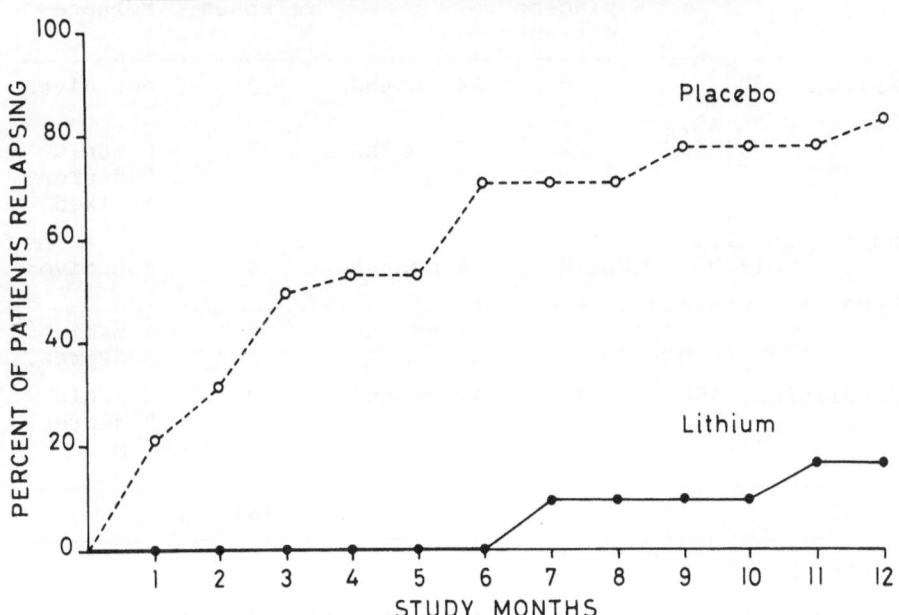

FIGURE 2 illustrates the cumulative frequency of relapses
          expressed in percents of relapsing patients over
          the 12 months period.

More than 50% of patients on placebo have an affective
relapse after 6 months of lithium withdrawal for none of
the patients on lithium treatment. These results are
almost identical to the one reported by Baastrup et al (5).

Table 3. Double blind lithium vs placebo controlled
          discontinuation studies in bipolar illness

Study	N° of placebo patients	Follow-up	N° of relapses	Type of relapse
Melia, 1970[4]	8	24 months	7	not given
Baastrup et al, 1970[5]	22	5 months	12	6 mania 5 depres. 1 mixed
Hullin et al, 1972[6]	8	6 months	4	not given
Fyro & Petterson, 1977[7]	9	8 months	9	6 mania 3 depres.
Mendlewicz, 1983[+]	14	12 months	12	3 mania 8 depres. 1 mixed
Total	61	5-24 months	44(72%)	

+ present investigation

The relapse rates observed in double blind lithium
discontinuation studies for bipolar patients on placebo
together with the results of the present study are reported
in Table 3.

Out of a total of 61 placebo bipolar patients, 44 (72%)
presented a major affective relapse. In our study the
number of placebo patients relapsing at the end of the
twelve months period is 12 (85%) for only 2 patients in
the lithium group (14%).

Our results do not need many comments. They clearly
demonstrate the prophylactic efficacy of long term lithium
treatment and the great risk of severe relapse even after
non abrupt lithium withdrawal in bipolar patients who were
considered lithium responders before discontinuing the
treatment. The question of the occurence of an acute
lithium withdrawal syndrome after lithium withdrawal can
not be considered by this investigation since the lithium
wash-out period was

conducted over a two weeks period. In conclusion, lithium discontinuation in bipolar patients who had clearly shown a benefit from the treatment should be strongly discouraged unless severe life threatening side effects appear during lithium maintenance.

REFERENCES

1. Spitzer R.L., Endicott J., Robbins E. (1978) Research diagnostic criteria : rationale and reliability. Archives General of Psychiatry, 35 : 773-782.
2. Hamilton M. (1960) A rating scale for depression. Journal of Neurology Neurosurgery and Psychiatry, 23 :56-62
3. Murphy D.L., Beigel A., Weingartner H., Bunney W.E.Jr. (1974) The quantitation of manic behavior. Pharmacopsychiat. 7 : 203-220.
4. Melia P.I. (1970) Prophylactic lithium : a double-blind trial in recurrent affective disorders. Br J Psychiatry, 116 : 621-624.
5. Baastrup P.C., Poulsen J.C., Schou M., Thomsen K., Amdisen A. (1970) Prophylactic lithium : double-blind discontinuation in manic-depressive disorders. Lancet ii, 326-330.
6. Hullin R.P., McDonald R., Allsopp M.N.E. (1972) Prophylactic lithium in recurrent affective disorders. Lancet ii, 1044-1046.
7. Fyro B., Petterson U. (1977) A double-blind study of the prophylactic effect of lithium in manic-depressive disease. Acta Psychiatr Scand Suppl 269 : 17-22.

11
Lithium treatment in schizoaffective patients

M. DEL ZOMPO, A. BOCCHETTA, C. BURRAI, M. MELIS AND G. U. CORSINI

INTRODUCTION

Schizoaffective Disorders : The classification of functional psychoses has tra-
ditionally been dichotomous since Kraepelin(1) proposed the division into two
major, mutually exclusive entities: dementia praecox, currently referred to as
schizophrenia, and manic-depressive insanity. The first was seen as inevitably
deteriorative, while the latter was seen as leading to recovery. However, the
psychiatric literature is replete with descriptions of psychoses with mixed
features, so that a plethora of names by various authors has resulted. The term
schizoaffective was first used by Kasanin in 1933, when he described nine patients with good premorbid functioning who developed acute psychoses with a mix-
ture of schizophrenic and affective symptoms and recovered after a few months
(2). Labeling this entity as schizoaffective was to focus on only a minority of
its features i.e. the acute symptom complex. Since then, therefore, there
has been a great deal of debate as to its meaning and validity (3) and it has
even been suggested that the term has created more mischief than it has resolved confusion (4). Anyhow, even contemporary trends in psychiatry reveal the
continued influence of the Kraeplinian dichotomy in the purpose of elucidating
the meaning of the concept "schizoaffective". The disagreement is whether
it is a subtype of schizophrenia, a subtype of affective disorder or a distinct
entity, and it is reflected in the DSM-III decision not to give operational
criteria for schizoaffective disorders (5). Thus a large number of cases is re-
legated to a mixed or atypical category and the diagnostic system cannot be
considered satisfactory in this regard. Unlike DSM-III, the Research Diagnostic
Criteria (RDC) by Spitzer et al (6) do have operational criteria for the schizoaffective disorders and have divided the syndrome into manic and depressive
type too. However, RDC have the problem of evaluating only the acute symptom
complex and not taking into account other factors needed for the schizoaffective state to be considered a valid diagnostic entity. In fact, we need additional data about epidemiology, including sex ratio and age of onset, premorbid
functioning, response to treatment, course of illness, family history and etiology with possible biological correlates. The importance of such factors
may be underlined by an example: the introduction of lithium salts treatment
has not only shown therapeutic implications but has also resulted in diagnostic
bias in favour of affective psychoses by American psychiatrists (7).

Treatment with Lithium salts.

The effectiveness of lithium treatment in schizoaffective patients is far from being assessed. There are numerous uncontrolled and controlled studies and several review articles on this subject, but no conclusion can be drawn. Most of the reports deal with short-term trials in the purpose of evaluating the efficacy of lithium in excited patients (8,9). Controlled studies have in general found neuroleptic treatment alone superior to lithium carbonate alone (10,11). Lithium salts have been reported to be effective only on hyperactivity and excitement whereas so-called core schizophrenic symptoms are unresponsive (12,13,14). On the other hand some Authors suggest that lithium carbonate has a modest but consistent beneficial effect as a supplement to neuroleptic treatment of the acute phase of excited schizoaffective illness. The positive effect is apparent in many symptoms and not specifically on purely "manic" ones such as euphoria or talkativeness (15). However, depressive schizoaffectives have not been included in such short-term studies and diagnostic criteria have generally focused on only acute symptom complex.

On the other hand, long-term studies carried out to evaluate a possible prophylactic benefit of lithium treatment for schizoaffectives are mostly uncontrolled (16,17) or include too few schizoaffectives (18,19). Moreover, they have often dealt with heterogeneous groups of patients due to previously discussed diagnostic problems; the nebulous term "improvement" has been too frequently used and the subjects' responses have not been clearly defined. An important task for future research is the more specific clarification of lithium responsive features using more homogeneous diagnostic criteria and taking into account the above mentioned additional data.

We have examined a group of patients diagnosed as manic or depressive schizo affectives according to RDC and with a follow-up of at least four years. We have also considered age of onset, prevalence of symptoms, premorbid adjustment, family history, course of illness and response to treatment, in order to evaluate the homogeneity of such patients according to both RDC and responsiveness to lithium.

PATIENTS AND METHODS

Twenty-nine schizoaffective patients under treatment for at least four years at the Lithium Clinic of the University of Cagliari, Italy, were studied. Diagnosis was performed at the time of admission to the clinic, according to RDC : patients who had shown symptoms suggestive of schizophrenia for at least one week during an episode of mania or depression were diagnosed as schizoaffectives of manic or depressive type, respectively (see Tables 1 and 2). Beyond the direct clinical observation and interview we collected additional data using both information obtained from relatives and clinical records. Patients admitted to long-term lithium treatment had invariably a clinical history of at least two years. We divided patients into bipolar and unipolar according to whether or not at least one previous episode had shown opposite affective polarity. Nevertheless, the bipolarity appeared in some instances during the episode which directly preceded admission.

RESULTS

Symptoms shown on admission are listed in Tables 1 and 2. Out of 29 patients 9 were depressive schizoaffectives and 20 manic schizoaffectives. No significant differences in symptoms appeared between the groups of unipolar and bipolar schizoaffectives: the distinction was based only on previous episodes of both polarities (10 out of 19 bipolars), previous episodes of polarity contrary to that shown on admission (4/19) and/or change of polarity during the episode preceding admission (7/19)

TABLE 1

SYMPTOMS RECORDED AMONG DEPRESSIVE SCHIZOAFFECTIVES ON ADMISSION.

	BIPOLAR n = 5	UNIPOLAR n = 4
DEPRESSIVE SYMPTOMS		
Depression or dysphoric mood	5	4
Poor appetite or weight loss	1	2
Sleep disturbance	3	2
Loss of energy and interest	3	3
Retardation	2	4
Feelings of guilt or self reproach	3	4
Suicidal thoughts or behaviour	2	1
Mute or poverty of speech	2	0
SCHIZOPHRENIC SYMPTOMS		
Thought disorder or disjointed speech	2	2
Blunted affect or emotional withdrawal	0	0
Delusion of being controlled	2	3
Hallucinations	2	1

Table 3 shows some features of unipolar and bipolar patients. Note the rather high percentage of patients with age of onset over 30 years old. No patient revealed personality deterioration. All but two presented a current episode lasting less than six months. No diagnosis of schizoaffectivity had been made in their clinical history, but this fact is related more to diagnostic inconsistencies than to different clinical features of their previous episodes: indeed, they had frequently received diagnoses such as atypical psychosis, atypical depression, schizophreniform syndrome. Treatment administered during the acute episode on admission is shown in Table 4. Lithium was administered alone or in combination with another treatment to most of the patients (23/29), both manic schizoaffectives (17/20) and depressive schizoaffectives (6/9). After at least four years of Lithium Clinic attendance, the current treatment was (Table 5): lithium alone in 11 out of 29, lithium in combination in 14 out of 29, while the remaining 4 received other medications. In detail, a point to be noted is that 12 out of 20 manic schizoaffectives required the combination of lithium with neuroleptics. Serum lithium levels were maintained between 0.6 - 1.0 mEq/l in all outpatients. The number of episodes before admission was particularly high in manic type and bipolar schizoaffectives: however, all groups took advantage of long-term lithium treatment (Table 6), with several instances of episode-free patients.

TABLE 2

SYMPTOMS RECORDED AMONG MANIC SCHIZOAFFECTIVES ON ADMISSION.

	BIPOLAR n = 14	UNIPOLAR n = 6
MANIC SYMPTOMS		
Euphoria	13	6
Irritability	5	3
Overactivity	8	2
Pressure of speech	7	3
Flight of ideas	5	2
Grandiosity	1	2
Decreased sleep	8	6
Distractibility	7	4
SCHIZOPHRENIC SYMPTOMS		
Thought disorder or disjointed speech	3	3
Blunted affect or emotional withdrawal	0	0
Delusion of being controlled	9	4
Hallucinations	6	2

TABLE 3

CHARACTERISTICS OF SCHIZOAFFECTIVE PATIENTS

	BIPOLAR n = 19	UNIPOLAR n = 10
Age of onset > 30	6	4
Familiarity	1	4
Previous psychiatric hospitalizations	15	8
Previous schizoaffective diagnoses	0	0
Duration of symptoms prior to admission		
less than 6 months	18	9
more than 6 months	1	1
Evidence of personality deterioration	0	0

TABLE 4

TREATMENT DURING EPISODE	DEPRESSIVE SCHIZOAFFECTIVES n = 9	MANIC SCHIZOAFFECTIVES n = 20
Lithium	2	2
Lithium + Neuroleptics	3	15
Lithium + Antidepressants	1	0
Neuroleptics	1	3
Neuroleptics + Antidepressants	1	0
Antidepressants	1	0

DISCUSSION

Our data are too preliminary to enable the drawing of definite conclusions about such controversial issue as schizoaffective disorders, but useful indications may arise from some points.

First, we underline the need for diagnostic criteria which take into account this condition, however it may be considered in relation to schizophrenia and manic-depressive psychosis. Our opinion is that RDC are reliable in order to obtain homogeneous groups of patients, even though based only upon clusters of acute symptoms. Thus, we suggest that the course of illness and the affective bipolarity, if any, should be further considered since previous reports have only marginally regarded this aspect.

TABLE 5

CURRENT TREATMENT IN SCHIZOAFFECTIVE OUTPATIENTS.	DEPRESSIVE ON ADMISSION n = 9	MANIC ON ADMISSION n = 20
Lithium	5	6
Lithium + Neuroleptics	1	12
Lithium + Antidepressants	1	0
Neuroleptics	0	2
Neuroleptics + Antidepressants	1	0
Antidepressants	1	0

TABLE 6

NUMBER OF EPISODES OF SCHIZOAFFECTIVE PATIENTS.

	BEFORE LITHIUM TREATMENT	DURING 4 YEARS OF LITHIUM TREATMENT
Unipolar Depressive	3 - 7	0 - 1
Bipolar (Depressive on admission)	2 - 16	0 - 3
Unipolar Manic	2 - 35	0 - 1
Bipolar (Manic on admission)	1 - 15	0 - 2

Shopsin for instance noted that classically these patients had an episode which displayed one pole of an affective illness and clear-cut schizophrenic symptoms which alternated with the other polar episode, which is indistinguishable from a pure affective illness (20). As already discussed, it may be difficult to diagnose schizoaffective disorder retrospectively, due to the inconsistencies of criteria used, nevertheless our patients seem to have shown previous episodes with already mixed, features according to diagnoses received. In any case, a rather high percentage (65%) had an affectively bipolar course. This may be an important point if one wishes to locate schizoaffective disorders in relation to major psychoses; moreover some literature suggests that manic schizoaffectives have the spectrum of bipolar illnesses in their families (21, 22, 23). Although family history data suffer even more from diagnostic problems, since they are frequently unclear, incomplete and based upon indirect information. Thus, our groups of patients are too small to give statistically significant indications about incidence of psychiatric illnesses in relatives, but to our knowledge, only five out of 29 patients had a positive family history. On the other hand, absence of personality deterioration, age of onset over 30 years old in one third of cases, and duration of symptoms before admission clearly distinguish our cases from schizophrenia. Course of illness, response to treatment and long-term outcome confirm this view, even though we must consider that one of our criteria of inclusion in the study was the attendance of the Clinic for four years after admission and we might have missed deteriorative patients. However, most of our schizoaffective outpatients (86%) benefit from long-term lithium treatment, as do manic-depressives, but it is noteworthy that a rather high percentage of manic schizoaffectives (60%) require supplemental neuroleptics, even though in small dosage, indicating that their condition is more severe than pure manic-depressive illness, whether or not we want to consider it a separate entity.

In conclusion, we suggest that schizoaffective disorders need serious consideration from different points of view: clinically it is of great importance to keep this in mind when treating and predicting outcome of patients with acute mixed symptoms. On the other hand, despite the longevity and abundance of specific literature, our understanding of this disorder is not clear. The lack of data concerning incidence in population is significant to this regard and is mostly due to the inclusion in schizophrenia or affective disorders according to the vogue in different times and countries. The use of specific diagnostic criteria and the evaluation of various dimensions would allow a clarification until the neurobiological basis of psychoses will be better known.

REFERENCES

1) Kraepelin E.: Dementia Praecox and Paraphrenia. Edinburgh, E&S Livingstone Ltd, 1919.
2) Kasanin J.: The acute schizoaffective psychoses. Am.J.Psychiatry 13, 97–126, 1933.
3) Klerman G.L., Barrett J.E.: The problem of schizoaffective states , In: Gershon S., Shopsin B. (eds.): Lithium: Its role in Psychiatric Research and Treatment. New York, Plenum Press Inc, 1973.
4) Batchelor I.R.C.: Henderson and Gillespie's Textbook of Psychiatry, ed.10, London, Oxford University Press, 1969.
5) American Psychiatric Association: Diagnostic and Statistical Manual of Mental Disorders, 3rd.Ed., American Psychiatric Association, Washington DC, 1981.
6) Spitzer R.L., Endicott J., Robins E.: Research Diagnostic Criteria, Ed.3, New York State Psychiatric Institute, 1977.
7) Baldessarini R.J.: Frequency of diagnosis of schizophrenia versus affective disorders from 1944 to 1968. Am.J.Psychiatry 127, 759–763, 1970.
8) Dinsmore P.R., Ryback R: Lithium in schizoaffective disorders. Dis.Nerv. Syst 33: 771–776, 1972.
9) Gleisinger B.: Evaluation of lithium treatment of psychotic excitement. Med. J.Aust. 41, 277–283, 1954.
10) Prien R.F., Caffey E.M., Klett C.J.: A comparison of lithium carbonate and chlorpromazine in the treatment of excited schizoaffectives. Arch.Gen.Psychiatry 27, 182–189, 1972.
11) Johnson G., Gershon S., Burdock E et al.: Comparative effects of lithium and chlorpromazine in the treatment of acute manic states. Br.J.Psychiatry 119, 267–276, 1971.
12) Schou M: Lithium in psychiatric therapy: Stock–taking after ten years. Psychopharmacologia 1, 65–78, 1959.
13) Gershon S., Yuwiler A.: Lithium ion: A specific psychopharmacological approach to the treatment of mania. J.Neuropsychiatry 1: 229–241, 1960.
14) Rimon R.: Lithium in the treatment of schizophrenia in: Psychiatrica Fennica 1973, Helsinki, Finland ,1973
15) Biederman J., Lerner Y., Belmaker R.H.: Combination of lithium carbonate and haloperidol in schizoaffective disorder. Arch.Gen.Psychiatry 36: 327–333, 1979.
16) Angst J.,Weis P., Grof.P. et al: Lithium prophylaxis in recurrent affective disorders. Br.J.Psychiatry 116: 604–614, 1970.
17) Perris C.: A study of cycloid psychoses. Acta Psychiatr.Scand, suppl.253, pp.1–74, 1974.
18) Melia P.L.: Prophylactic lithium: A double–blind trial in recurrent affective disorders. Br.J.Psychiatry 116: 621–624, 1970.
19) Prien R.F., Caffey E.M., Klett J.: Factors associated with treatment success in lithium carbonate prophylaxis. Arch.Gen.Psychiatry 31: 189–192, 1974.
20) Shopsin B.: Part 1 : Mania: Clinical aspects, rating scales and incidence of manic–depressive illness. In: Manic Illness, Shopsin B. (ed.), Raven Press, New York, 1979.

21) Abrams R., Taylor M.: Mania and schizoaffective disorder, manic type: A comparison . Am.J.Psychiatry 133: 1445–1447, 1976.

22) Rosenthal N.E., Rosenthal L.N., Stallone F.et al: Toward the validation of RDC schizoaffective disorder. Arch.Gen.Psychiatry 37: 804–810, 1980.

23) Pope H.G., Lipinski J.F., Cohen B.M. et al:"Schizoaffective disorder": an invalid diagnosis? A comparison of schizoaffective disorder, schizophrenia and affective disorder. Am.J.Psychiatry 137: 921–927, 1980.

12
Static and kinetic study of the RBC/plasma lithium ratio in manic-depressive, schizoaffective and schizophrenic patients in thymic remission: significance for diagnosis and monitoring

P. DENIKER, H. LOO, J.P. OLIE, C. GAY, C. BENKELFAT AND P. BINET

For the last few years, many clinical investigators have tried to prove that the lithium intraglobular determination is to be preferred to plasma lithium determination for monitoring lithium treatment.

The value of RBC/plasma lithium ratio as a diagnostic and pronostic aid as well as for predicting the therapeutic response remains a controversial issue.

The interest aroused by the in vivo RBC/plasma lithium ratio has given rise to many clinical studies. The normal range of values is between 0,2 and 1. Several parameters were described as capable of modifying this value, e.g. : age (1), sex (2), treatment (3), diagnosis or pathologic state (4,5,6), high blood pressure (7), alcoholism (8), obesity (9), renal insufficiency (10), H.L.A. system (11)...

Some authors have considered it a valuable biological marker for the differentiation of subgroups of depressive patients (2,12) while others have laid emphasis on its therapeutical value for predicting response to treatment (13, 14).

Adress reprint requests to : Pr. P. DENIKER, Service Hospitalo-Universitaire de Santé Mentale et de Thérapeutique, Hôp. Sainte-Anne, 1 rue Cabanis 75014 PARIS.

The present study discusses the kinetic of this lithium ratio in patients on long-term lithium treatment.

METHODS

·The study we present here was conducted in the service de Santé Mentale et de Thérapeutique (Pr DENIKER) for about 6 months at the end of 1981.

1) Subjects :

- All the 51 patients included in this study gave informed consent and had been treated with lithium treatment for more than 15 days. The study was performed at the end of hospitalisation and most of the patients were free of dysthymic symptoms. There were 16 women and 35 men and ages ranged from 23 to 68.

- The diagnoses met the DSM III criteria (15) and are distributed as follows :

  . major affective bipolar disorders (n = 25)
  . recurrent major depression (n = 4)
  . schizoaffective disorders (n = 14) corresponding to DSM III classification : 295-70
  . schizophrenia (n = 8).

- The 51 patients were allotted to subgroups according to diagnosis, drug combinations and clinical tolerance to lithium treatment.

- Several physiological parameters (sex, age, bodyweight) and therapeutical ones (daily dosage of the lithium salt, drug combination) were taken into account.

- The participants in the study were authorized to ingest only psychotropics (neuroleptics and/or benzodiazepines and/or antidepressants) and corrector of the psychotropic side effects (antiparkinsonian drugs, cardiovascular analeptics).

- None of the patients showed high blood pressure (Diastolic ≤ 95 mm Hg) or an abnormal kidney function (creatinine clearance ≥ 80 ml/mn; blood urea ≤ 8 mMl/l; absence of proteinuria).

2) Methodology

At 7 a.m., each patient took orally, in a single intake, the daily dose of lithium carbonate in order to keep serum lithium within the therapeutic range (tablet of 250 mg).

9 blood samples were drawn over 13 hours, the first one being taken immediately before lithium administration.

3) Analytic procedure

Lithium plasma and intra-erythrocytic levels were measured by the method described by Binet et all. (risk of error $\pm$ 0,05 mEq/l) (16).

- Blood sampling
  . 5 ml of venous blood drawn into a tube with anticoagulant without Li.
  . Centrifugation : 4000 R VS/mn - 15'.

- Determination plasma Li.
  . Flame photometry, (dilution 1/10)
  . Atomic Absorption SpectroPhotometry (dilution 1/1000) compared to suitable prepared standards (KCL).

- Determination of Erythrocyte-Li
  . Flame Photometry (Trichloroacétic extraction and dilution 1/50)
  . Atomic Absorption Spectrophotometry (Trichloroacetic extraction and dilution 1/5).

4) Statistics

- Static comparison of means of the RBC/plasma Li ratios in different subgroups according to the sex, age, weight, posology, diagnosis by student test.

- Kinetic comparison of means of RBC/plasma Li ratios at different times of the day in 2 subgroups according to tolerance = student test.

<u>RESULTS</u>

1) <u>Static study of some interindividual factors of variability</u> :

The value of lithium ratio obtained at 7 a.m. (i.e. twelve hours after the last dose) was not influenced by the various parameters studied.

a) <u>Sex</u>

- 16 females : lithium ratio = 0.433 ± 0.151
- 35 males   : lithium ratio = 0.481 ± 0.09

(no significant difference)

b) <u>Age</u> : <u>Influence of age on the Li ratio</u>

AGE	N	LI RATIO	
20 - 30	10	$0,49 \pm 0,10$	
31 - 40	18	$0,45 \pm 0,12$	
41 - 50	12	$0,48 \pm 0,14$	Table 1
51 - 60	7	$0,44 \pm 0,09$	
61 - 70	3	$0,44 \pm 0,07$	
71 - 80	1	$0,53 \pm 0,05$	

There was no significant difference found between the six age-groups studied.

c) <u>Bodyweight</u>

WEIGHT	N	LI RATIO	
41 - 50	3	$0,60 \pm 0,13$	
51 - 60	7	$0,42 \pm 0,09$	
61 - 70	18	$0,50 \pm 0,09$	Table 2
71 - 80	15	$0,42 \pm 0,11$	
81 - 90	5	$0,48 \pm 0,14$	
91 - 100	3	$0,36 \pm 0,12$	

There was no significant difference found in the mean values of Li-ratio according to bodyweight with the exception of the last weight-group that included only three patients : in these cases, the Li-ratio value tended to be lower.

d) Dosage

Different doses were given to seven groups of patients. No difference was seen in lithium ratio values between the patients groups.

Influence of Li Daily-dose on Li ratio

DAILY DOSE	N	LI RATIO	
250 mg	1	0,53 + 0,05	
500 mg	3	0,34 + 0,16	
750 mg	10	0,45 ÷ 0,07	
1000 mg	14	0,47 ÷ 0,13	Table 3
1250 mg	16	0,49 + 0,11	
1500 mg	5	0,45 ÷ 0,16	
1750 mg	2	0,45 ÷ 0,06	

e) Diagnosis

Finally there was no difference in the Li-ratio values obtained
in the various diagnostic groups at the time of Normothymia. The
study was not longitudinal so we did not compare lithium ratio values
between pathological state and thymic remission.

The mean Li-ratio values at zero time (i.e. twelve hours after
le last dose) were calculated for each diagnostic subgroup (table 4).

Dg	N	PLASMA LI	RBC LI	PLASMA LI-RATIO
Manic Depressive Bipolar 296 - 5 X	25	0,75 + 0,22	0,36 + 0,13	0,42 ÷0,12
Manic Depressive Unipolar 296 - 3 X	4	0,74 + 0,9	0,36 + 0,03	0,49 ÷ 0,07
Schizo-Affective Disorder 295 - 70	14	0,75 ÷ 0,16	0,35 + 0,1	0,49 ± 0,1
Schizophrenia 295 - XX	8	0,78 + 0,13	0,32 + 0,1	0,43 ÷0,12

2) <u>Kinetic diurnal study of the RBC plasma Li-ratio</u>

We observed a high intrapatient variation in Li-ratio values.

In some cases, this diurnal variation was as high as 130 %. In the

51 patients the mean Li-ratio values was 0.394 $\div$ 0.10 at 9 a.m. and

0.516 at 4 p.m. and the difference was significant at P<0.0001.

(student test) The 2 curves illustrate this   point.

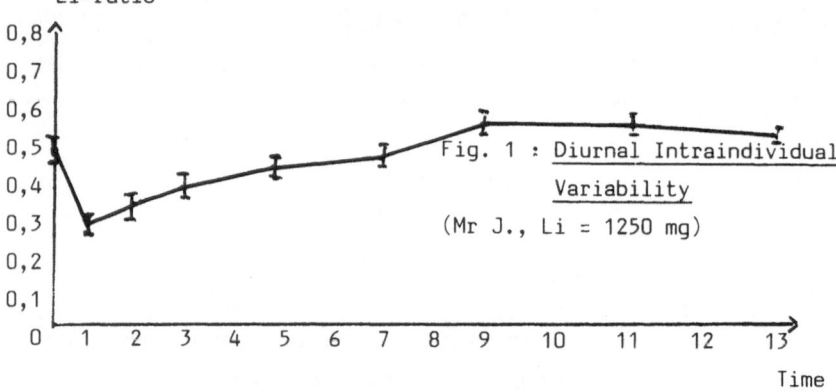

Fig. 1 : <u>Diurnal Intraindividual</u>

<u>Variability</u>

(Mr J., Li = 1250 mg)

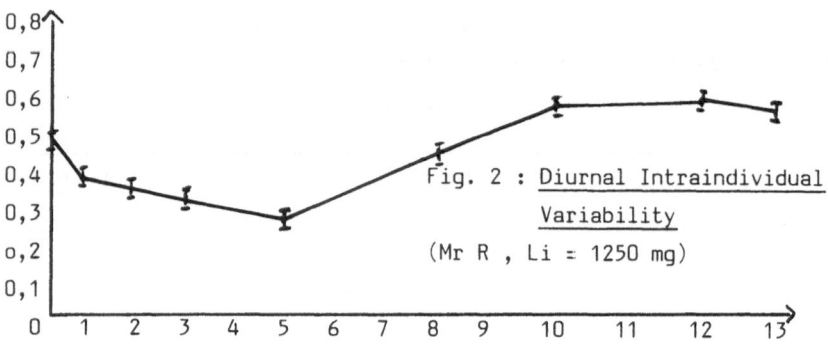

Fig. 2 : <u>Diurnal Intraindividual</u>

<u>Variability</u>

(Mr R , Li = 1250 mg)

They represent the values obtained in two male patients age 40 and
50 who have reached a steady state with 1250 mg of lithium carbonate.
The first curve shows a marked reduction of the lithium ratio during
the first hour, probably due to the sudden increase in plasma lithium,
then a gradual increase in Li-ratio related to the secondary passage
of lithium into the red blood cell. The second curve shows a similar
profile which however is more pronounced.

These two examples illustrate the intraindividual variability of the
Li-ratio during the day. It corresponds to normally expected
pharmacokinetic data.

However, this is well above a risk of error which is negligible if
one considers a measurement point reflecting a moment in the
kinetic evolution of the lithium ion.

- Li-ratio and Neurological tolerance to treatment.

We considered also in this study 2 subgroups of patients according
to good or poor neurological tolerance to lithium treatment.
The manifestations selected as signs of neurological intolerance
to treatment with the lithium salts ranged from slight tremors of the
extremity to the obvious picture of full-blown intoxication, mental
confusion and spasmodic muscular contractions.

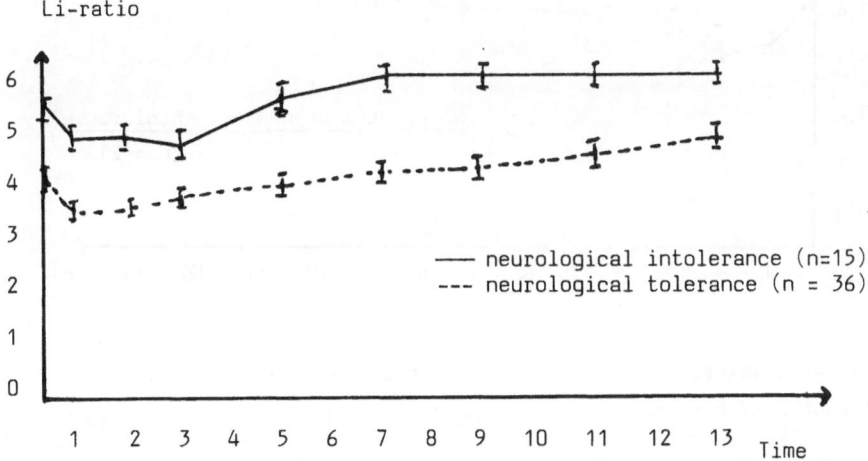

Fig. 3 : Li-ratio and Neurological tolerance to treatment

- In conformity with this description, 36 patients were considered
lithium tolerant as they showed no side-effects while 15 were intolerant.

The Li-ratio value was significantly higher in lithium-intolerant
than in lithium-tolerant patients (Fig. 3). Nevertheless, kinetic
curves for tolerant and intolerant patients were parallel.

The increased Li-ratio values in intolerant patients corresponded
to an increased RBC lithium with inchanged plasma concentration.

- 21 tolerant and 13 intolerant patients received a lithium-
phenothiazine combination

Figure 4 : <u>Neurological intolerance to lithium : possible role
of Li-Phenothiazine combination.</u>

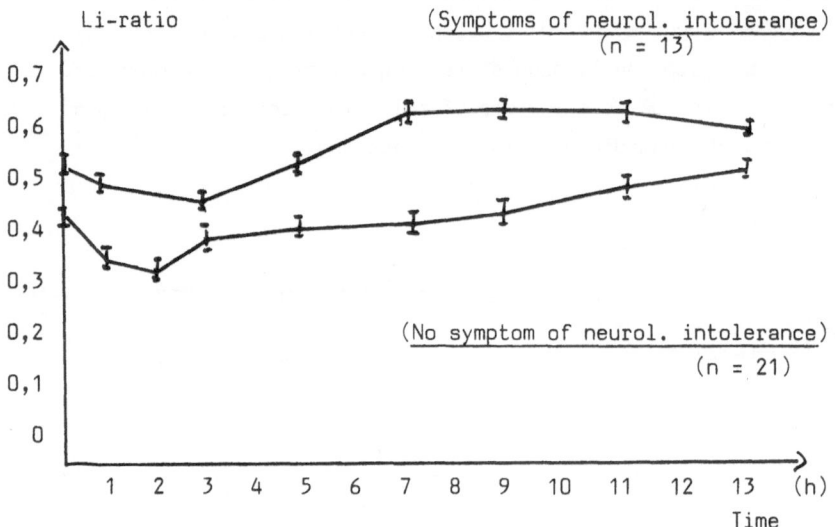

Li-ratio values were significantly higher in intolerant than in
tolerant patients whatever the sampling time (p > 0.01).

DISCUSSION

The present work on RBC/plasma lithium kinetics in 51 patients made
it possible to demonstrate the following findings.

. No difference in RBC/plasma ratios was found in the various
subgroups of patients according to age, sex, weight, dosage and
diagnosis.

. In contrast, marked intraindividual diurnal variations were
observed : minimum and maximum values were found 2 and 9 hours after
lithium ingestion. Therefore this index is difficult to interpret.

. There was no difference in plasma lithium levels between tolerant
and intolerant patients but in contrast a positive correlation was
seen to exist between RBC lithium levels and manifestations of intolerance to lithium therapy.

These results are consistent with clinical studies wich have
s hown a relationship between increased lithium ratio and toxic effects
observed when lithium blood levels were within the therapeutic range
(17, 18). In contrast withfindings of others (19) no relationship was
found between the incidence of i ntolerance manifestations and schizophrenia diagnosis, may be because of the small number of patients.

. In the present study a large percentage of intolerant patients
received lithium and phenothiazine derivatives and had a high lithium
ratio. Lithium-phenothiazine combination has been repeatedly found to
be responsible for neurotoxic effects (20, 21, 22).

RBC lithium increase may be ascribed to phenothiazine action on
the cell membrane (3). Phenothiazine derivatives increase passive
permeability to cations. However, no difference was seen between
tolerant patients given lithium alone and tolerant patients given
lithium-phenothiazine combination.

The hypothesis of a facilitating action of phenothiazines should
be corroborated by an in vivo study of phenothiazine action on lithium
transport across the red cell membrane. A number of parameters including phenothiazine and lithium plasma concentrations, passive permeability regulatory systems (ATP, membrane and plasma lipids...) and
treatment duration should be taken into account in such study.

The following question could also be answered by a study of this type : is the in vitro increase in the passive permeability to lithium induced by phenothiazine, observed in vivo ?

CONCLUSION

Kinetic investigation of lithium revealed the intrapatient variations (variability) in RBC/plasma lithium ratio.

A correlation was found between the increase in the lithium level in red blood cells (and consequently that of the lithium ratio) and clinical manifestations of intolerance.

Future work will have to determine wether clinical intolerance to lithium biologically proved by a raise of RBC/plasma lithium ratio is to be attributed to a drug combination which favors the accumulation of the lithium within the red blood cells or to a particular predisposition of some patients to accumulate lithium within their red blood cells. Other factors could be invoked.

The diagnosis value of the RBC/plasma lithium ratio was not demonstrated in the present study : no relation was found between lithium ratio and any nosologic classification.

Should the predisposition be confirmed, the RBC/plasma lithium ratio would be a valuable contribution to the detection of subgroups of high-risk patients.

BIBLIOGRAPHY

1. ALBRECHT J., MULLER-OERLINGHAUSEN B. (1976)
   Clinical relevance of lithium determination in RBC : results of a
   catamnestic study.
   Arzneim Forsch, 26, 1145-1147.

2. LITKENS L., SODERBERG U., WETTERBERG L. (1973)
   Increased lithium erythrocyte plasma ratio in manic depressive
   psychosis.
   Lancet, 1, 40.

3. PANDEY G.N., GOEL I., DAVIS JM. (1979)
   Effects of neuroleptic drugs on lithium uptake by human
   erythrocyte.
   Clin. Pharmacol. Ther., 26, 96-102.

4. ELIZUR A., SHOPSIN B., GERSHON S., EHLENBERGER A. (1972)
   Intra/extra cellular lithium ratios and clinical course in
   affective states.
   Clin. Pharmacol. Ther., 13, 947-952.

5. MENDELS J., FRAZER A. (1974)
   Alteration in cell membrane activity in depression.
   Am. J. Psychiatry, 131, 1240-1246.

6. RYBAKOWSKI J. (1977)
   Pharmacogenetic aspect of red blood cell lithium index in manic-
   depressive psychosis.
   Biol. Psychiatry, 12, (3), 425-429.

7. CANESSA M., ADRAGNA N., SOLOMON H.S., CONOLLY J.M., TOSTESON D.C.
   (1980)
   Increased sodium-lithium countertransport in red cells of patients
   with essential hypertension.
   In N. England J. Med., 302, (14), 772-776.

8. GUERRI C., RIBELLES M., GRISOLIA S. (1981)
   Effects of lithium and lithium and alcohol administration on
   (NA^+K^+) Pomp.
   In "Biochemical Pharmacology", Vol 30, pp 25-30.

9. DE LUISE M., BLACBURN G.L., FLIER J.S. (1980)
   Reduced activity of the red-cell sodium-potassium pump in human
   obesity.
   In "The New-England J. of Med." 303, (18), 1017-1022.

10. BAASTRUUP P.C. (1979)
    Absolute and relative conterindications for prophylactic
    lithium treatment.
    In Lithium : contreversis and unresolved issues.
    Edit : T.B. COOPER, S. GERSHON, N.S. KLINE, M. SCHOV.
    Exerpta Medica, Amsterdam, Oxford, PRINCETON, pp 413-418.

11. SMERALDI E., SCORZA-SMERALDI R., CAZZULLO C.L. (1979)
    HLA System and Psychopharmacology.
    In "Biological Psychiatry Today". J. OBIOLS, C. BALLUS,
    E. GONZALES MONCLUS, J. PUJOL eds.
    ELSEVIER/NORD Holland Biomedical Press, Amsterdam.

12. LYTTEKENS L., S'ODERBERG, WETTERBERG L.(1976)
    Relation between erythrocyte and plasma lithium concentrations
    as an index in psychiatric disease.
    Ups. J. Med. Sci., 131, 1240-1246.

13. CASPER R.C., PANDEY G., GOSENFELD L., DAVIS JM. (1976)
    Intra cellular lithium and clinical response.
    Lancet, 2,,418-419.

14. GREIL W., EISENRIED F., BECKER BF., DUHM J. (1977)
    Interindividual differences in the Na^+ dependent Li^+ counter
    transport system and in the Li^+ distribution ratio across the
    red cell membrane among Li^+ treated patients.
    Psychopharmacology, 53, 19-26.

15. AMERICAN PSYCHIATRIC ASSOCIATION Committee on nomenclature and
    statistics. (1980)
    Diagnostic and statistical manual of mental disorders.
    3rd Edition, Washington, DC : American Psychiatric Association.

16. BINET P., LY R., JEAN LOUIS J. (1981)
    Dosage du lithium plasmatique et globulaire par photométrie de
    flamme.
    Détermination du rapport érythrplasmatique.
    Pharm. Biol., 15, 221-225.

17. DYSKEN MW., COMATY JE., PANDEY GN., DAVIS JM. (1979)
    Asterixis associated with a high RBC lithium concentration.
    Am. J. Psychiatry, 136, 1610.

18. OLIE JP., GAY C., LOO H., ZARIFIAN E., POIRIER-LITTRE MF.,
    DENIKER P. (1982)
    L'intérêt du dosage du lithium intra-érythrocytaire dans la
    surveillance bioclinique de la lithiothérapie.
    Ann. Biol. Clin., 40, 3-10.

19. SHOPSIN B.,KIM S., GERSHON S. (1971)
    A controlled study of lithium vs chlorpormazine in acute
    schizophrenics.
    Br. J. Psychiat., 119, 435-440.

20. BOUDOURESQUES G., PONCET M., ALI CHERIF A., TAGANI B.,
    BOUDOURESQUES L. (1980)
    Encéphalopathie aigue au cours d'un traitement associant
    phénothiazine et lithium.
    Nouv. Press. Med., 9, 2580.

21. BRACCINI T., COAT C., LAVAGNA J., MYQUEL M., DARCOURT G.
    Tolérance neurologique de l'association lithium-psychotropes.
    A partir de 265 cures associatives.
    Encéphale, 7, 29.

22. SPRING GK. (1979)
    Neurotoxicity with combined use of lithium and thioridazine.
    J. Clin. Psychiatry, 40, 135.

Acknowledgements : *We greatly appreciate the skillful technical
assistance of all nurses who participate to this study.*
This present paper has been submitted for publication to "THERAPIE"

13
Lithium prophylaxis in major affective disorders: on the specificity and sensitivity of some "new" predictors of treatment outcome

E. SACCHETTI, A. VITA, G. CONTE AND A. PENNATI

INTRODUCTION

Since the controversy over the long term efficacy of lithium has been definitively overcome with the unequivocal
demonstration that lithium is a valuable treatment for
both the prevention and the attenuation of affective recurrences in a substantial portion of patients suffering
from Major Affective Disorders (MAD) (1,2,3), studies
with lithium have been focused more and more on attempts
to predict which candidates might be expected to have
good lithium responses (4,5,6,7). Clinical and experimental
needs both require this type of research. First of all,
adequate recognition of patients who will respond differently to lithium, not only gives a rational basis for
whether or not to undertake long term lithium stabilization,
it also influences investigations of new putative stabilizing treatments (8), since the definition of the risk-benefit
ratios of these alternative therapies will weigh differently if they are chiefly indicated for lithium responders
or lithium non-responders. Furthermore, the differentiation
of lithium responders from lithium non-responders could

be of fundamental importance for proper understanding of the basic processes underlying the disease in the different subgroups of MAD.

For all these reasons, we have been engaged for some years in a search for possible predictors of long term lithium effectiveness. Since an enlarged body of evidences demonstrates that MAD is a disease with an intrinsic biological heterogeneity (9,10,11,12,13,14,15), after initial attempts (6,7,16,17) to predict by means of para- meters quite different from the indices usually utilized for individuate meaningful subgroups among MAD patients, we have found it more appropriate to predict chiefly from variables which seem to cluster patients into independent groups, each with its own peculiar and distinct internal characteristics.

In this presentation, our recent and present studies in this area will be summarized, with especial attention to the issues of the specificities and sentivities of the different putative predictors we have tested.

SAMPLE AND PROCEDURE

The patients studied in the separate experimental protocols add up to 105 (49 men, 56 women), with a mean age of 47.3 at the moment when long term lithium prophylaxis was started. At admission all the patients fully met the criteria for primary affective disorders (18) and, retrospectively, those for MAD (19); 57 were subclassified as bipolar and 48 as unipolar. The occurrence of two or more affective episodes in the two years immediately preceding lithium prophylaxis and a history of at least four episodes since the onset of the disease were addit- ional required criteria for inclusion. The patients select ed by this procedure have been systematically seen at least once a month by experienced psychiatrists in the Research Unit for Affective Disorders of the Institute of Clinical Psychiatry of Milan Medical School. At the same times, blood samples were taken for plasma lithium levels and the lithium doses adjusted individually to maintain plasma lithium levels between 0.6 and 0.95 mmol/L 12 hours after the last dose. Once a year the patients were also checked for possible toxic lithium effects. The periods of follow up during lithium treatment ranged from 32 to 64 months, with a mean of 52 ± 8 (SD) months.

At the end of this follow up the patients were classified as good or poor responders without knowledge of the different variables being analyzed as possible predictors of lithium outcome. The criterion of classification was whether or not, during the time period between 8 months after the initiation of lithium prophylaxis and the end of the follow up, there had been at least one major affective episode requiring supplementary medication with antidepressants or neuroleptics plus carbamazepine. This selection procedure was chosen on the basis that it is not only easy to apply and less influenced by subjective evaluation but, also, because it is very restrictive in its definition of a good lithium responder and would not include an appreciable number of false poor lithium responders. In fact, of the large sample of patients actually followed at the Research Unit, over 78% of the patients classified as lithium non-responders have had multiple affective breakdowns (20), and specifically considering the population under examination, none of the poor lithium responders had single recurrences during lithium prophylaxis.

Our population had an overall rate of 52% of good lithium responses. Values discordant with this in the separate studies are due to the fact that some patients were studied under more than one protocol and others under only one.

The lack of any discernible differences between responders and non-responders in either the number of affective recurrences per year before starting lithium prophylaxis or the mean plasma lithium levels seems to exclude the idea that differences in lithium outcome might have been due to the fact that the group of poor lithium responders have a more severe form of the disease or received inadequate lithium dosages.

MHPG AND AGE OF ONSET

The bulk of evidence obtained in studies of different indices of monoamine (MA) turnover is undoubtedly the best proof that MAD is heterogeneous, with subgroups of patients with rather specific clinical and pharmacological characterization being recognizable whatever biochemical parameter is studied (9,10,11,12,13,15,21).

On the basis of urinary MHPG excretion data, MAD can be divided into two basic archetypes, one with high and one with low MHPG excretion, which differ from each other not only in the age of onset (6,21,22,23) and possibly in the proclivity to develop mania (9,10,12,15,21, 22,23) but also, although it is still controversial, in the responsiveness to various antidepressants (9,10,11, 12,13,15,21,24,25). Therefore we started to look for the relationship between response to long term lithium treatment and urinary MHPG (26).

Since it is not yet definitively established whether urinary MHPG is a state or a trait-dependent variable (for references: 12), we utilized the MHPG values during depressive phases, postulating that they should in any case express differences in the biological background also operating more or less subliminally during the non-depressive phase of the disease. Furthermore since age, age of onset of the disease, its duration and polarity and the sex of the patient seem not to be completely independent of either the urinary MHPG (6,9,10,12,13,15,21,22,23) or the natural prognosis of MAD (4,27,28), all of these variables were also taken into account and included in a stepwise regression analysis with long term lithium outcome as the dependent variable.

The analysis for 25 bipolar patients (26) showed a very high cumulative power of the set of the independent variables for predicting the subsequent outcome during lithium prophylaxis: 68% of the total variance was, in fact, accounted for and the multiple correlation was 0.83. Almost all the correlation appeared to be due to urinary MHPG and age of onset, which had inverse partial correlations of 0.85 and 0.26. The other factors were found to be substantially without effect.

The analysis for 24 unipolar patients (26) gave less striking, but not negligible, results in the same direction: all the independent variables had in fact a multiple correlation of 0.39, which expresses a 15% cumulative control of the variance. In this case too, MHPG and age of onset weighed more than the other variables, with inverse simple correlations of 0.35 and 0.24. Corrections for interactions showed, however, that the apparent effect of age of onset was due to a second order association, since this variable accounted per se for only 25% of the variance. In light of this, age of onset was not used in subsequent analyses. The lack of power of MHPG to differentiate lithium responders and lithium non-responders within a population of unipolar patients was chiefly due to excessive fluctuations among the lithium non-responders of the parameters investigated. The MHPG values of non-responders were, in fact, quite evenly distributed over the entire range found in MAD patients, while only one lithium responder was a high MHPG excretor.

The results of these two stepwise regression analyses shed some light on the pleiotropic effect of the drug-patient interaction and permit us to infer the mechanisms that may be responsible for the stabilizing effects of lithium. They seem to strengthen the idea that there are pathogenetically distinct subgroups of MAD patients. Nevertheless, the information is less applicable when we are dealing with single patients and must decide whether or not treat them prophylactically with lithium. In this situation, careful estimation of the probability of erroneous prediction for that specific individual is more relevant than a precise quantification of the specific predictive power of a given variable within a group of patients.

For this reason, the specificity and sensitivity of MHPG and age of onset for selecting different lithium outcomes were tested in an enlarged sample. Binary grouping criteria - definitely low (less than 1600 μg/24hrs) versus definitely high (more than 2000 μg/24hrs) MHPG values and definitely early (less than 38 years) versus definitely late (more than 42 years) onsets, with high

MHPG and, for bipolars only, late age of onset as indices of poor lithium responsiveness - were therefore utilized instead of the continuous values employed in the earliear stepwise regression analyses.

For bipolar patients MHPG (Table 1) predicted different lithium outcomes with extreme precision (95.7%), with both specificity and sensitivity impressively high (100% and 91%).

Table 1. Urinary MHPG and lithium outcome in bipolars.

Specificity	100%	False positives	-
Sensitivity	91%	False negatives	4.3%
	Correct prediction	95.7%	

Age of onset gave a somewhat increased rate of errors of classification (41.3%); misclassifications appeared to be chiefly due to false negatives - i.e., patients with early onset and poor lithium outcome - since together with fully satisfactory specificity (83%), the sensitivity was relatively low (50%) (Table 2).

Table 2. Age of onset and lithium outcome in bipolars.

Specificity	83%	False positives	4.3%
Sensitivity	50%	False negatives	37 %
	Correct prediction	58.7%	

For unipolar patients, MHPG (Table 3) led to correct selection in 71.5% of the cases; false positives and false negatives contributed to the lower predictive value than that for bipolar patients in an unbalanced way, with the effects of false negatives predominating: in fact, while the specificity of high MHPG as a predictor of poor lithium responsiveness was noteworthy (85.6%) for unipolar patients too, the sensitivity was less good (65.6%), since almost 23.7% of low MHPG excretors in our sample relapsed.

Table 3. Urinary MHPG and lithium outcome in unipolars.

Specificity	85.6%	False positives	4.8%
Sensitivity	64.4%	False negatives	23.7%
	Correct prediction	71.5%	

These results extend to clinical practice the findings of eminently theoretical relevance acquired in the previous stepwise analyses (26): they clearly indicate that both MHPG and age of onset may be valid practical tools which may help the clinician by increasing his ability to predict ahead of time what will happen during lithium maintainance therapy. In this connection, it should be further emphasized that high MHPG levels do seem to predict poor lithium responses in bipolar patients with the same precision as low MHPG levels predict good lithium responses. On the contrary, age of onset in bipolar patients and MHPG in unipolar patients are not so consistently predictive, since high MHPG and late age of onset appear to be able to identify poor lithium responders better than low MHPG and early age of onset identify good lithium responders.

TRICYCLIC ANTIDEPRESSANT DRUGS

Independent evidence agrees that individual pharmacological profiles for tricyclic antidepressant drugs (TADs) may be a useful but operatively rather neglected tool for categorizing MAD patients into more homogeneous subgroups. MAD patients seem to have stable responses to the various TADs: responders to a given TAD during a depressive episode are generally benefited by the same treatment in the subsequent episodes and patients who do not improve on a given TAD can be predicted not to respond to the same treatment in future episodes (29), even when an adequate dose of a drug is given (30). Furthermore, it appears that the response to one TAD predicts the quality of the response to other TADs, with indications for amitriptyline (AMI) and clomipramine (CLOMI) largely overlapping and quite different from those for nortriptyline (NTP) and desipramine (DMI) (21,31). Finally, suggestions (21,31) of a possible and stable linkage with time between individual pharmacological profiles and the individual biochemical patterns of the MAD fit well with these clinical observations and give some biological substantiation to these findings.

With the aim of having a preordered non-instrumental foundation for classifying subgroups of patients, each with a putative different prognosis on lithium prophylaxis, it seemed therefore of value to also utilize their previous pharmacological histories on the TADs (32). Evidence for some relationship between MHPG and responses to both TADs (9,10,11,12,13,15,21,24,25) and lithium (26) would theoretically be a bridge between the two.

The analysis of 40 cases treated with AMI (1.2 - 2 mg/Kg/day) showed a non-chance relationship between clinical response to this antidepressant drug and long term effectiveness. In fact, 8 of 11 poor responders to AMI had good lithium outcomes while only 8 of 29 good responders to AMI were succesfully treated prophylactically with lithium (chi square = 5.02; p < .05).

Similar results were obtained with 30 CLOMI-treated patients; it was evident that there is a higher frequency of lithium non-responders among CLOMI responders (20 of 24) than among CLOMI non-responders (2 of 6) (chi square = 3.846; p < .05). The prediction of long term lithium effectiveness by means of previous responses to AMI and CLOMI (Table 4 and 5) was correct for 72.5% of the cases treated with the first drug and for 80% of the cases treated with the second drug and the criteria "good response to AMI or to CLOMI - poor lithium outcome" had similar specificities (72% and 83%) and sensitivities (73% and 67%).

Table 4.Response to AMI and lithium outcome in MAD patients.

Specificity	72%	False positives	20 %
Sensitivity	73%	False negatives	7.5%
	Correct prediction	72.5%	

There were inverse associations for the NTP - and DMI-treated patients. Responders to NTP were satisfactorily protected by lithium against affective recurrences at

Table 5.Response to CMI and lithium outcome in MAD patients.

Specificity	83%	False positives	13.3%
Sensitivity	67%	False negatives	13.3%
		Correct prediction	80%

---

a higher rate than NTP non-responders (21 of 31 vs 1 of 13 cases) (chi square = 10.91; p < .001). Therefore the criterion "good response to NTP" as a predictor for good lithium response (Table 6) had a specificity of 68% and a sensitivity of 92% and permitted correct prediction of lithium outcome for 75% of the cases.

Table 6.Response to NTP and lithium outcome in MAD patients.

Specificity	68%	False positives	22.7%
Sensitivity	92%	False negatives	2.3%
		Correct prediction	75%

In an analogous way, although the size of the sample was clearly too small - 16 subjects - for more than an exploration, classification of patients according to their responses to DMI separated lithium responders from lithium non-responders for 83.4% of the cases: DMI-responders were more prone to good lithium outcomes (5 of 7) than DMI non-responders, who were always lithium non-responders, so that the association of good responses to both DMI and lithium apparently had a specificity of 72% and a sensitivity of 100% (Table 7).

Table 7.Response to DMI and lithium outcome in MAD patients.

Specificity	72%	False positives	16.6%
Sensitivity	100%	False negatives	-
		Correct prediction	83.4%

According to the independent comparisons, it seems there-fore that characterizations of patients according to their responses to TADs may be a valid, easy and non-time-consum-ing way to separate subgroups of patients with different clinical courses on lithium.

Though this paradigm seems apparently to be equally true for all four TADs, different interpretations can be formulated to justify the false positives and false negatives encountered from time to time when utilizing the response to any given antidepressant as a predictor of lithium outcome. First of all, unexpected good lithium responders among the NTP and DMI non-responders could be considered to be misclassifications due to inadequate dose regimens. Since their incidence was almost negligible, between 0 and 2.3% of non-responders to these two TADs, it can be inferred, generalizing also to the other TADs, that adequate doses of the antidepressants have probably been given to most of the patients. On this basis, only a small fraction of poor responders to both lithium and AMI or CMI can be in theory connected by such an interpre-tation. For most of the patients of this group, factors extraneous to the lithium outcome - TAD responsiveness relationship, but possibly related to some peculiarities inherent to lithium therapy should be more correctly taken into account. In analogy, these same factors unrelated to TADs might cause the few poor lithium outcomes encountered among NTP and/or DMI responders. A substantial number of the AMI or CMI responders who also benefited from lithium might have been due to an _in vivo_ conversion of these drugs to their secondary amines, which have spectra of biochemical activity quite unlike those of the parent compound. This is supported by independent findings that two of three responders to both lithium and CMI whose TAD plasma levels were measured had desmethylclomipramine levels higher than 100 ng/ml and 3 of 4 AMI responders who were satisfactorily stabilized by lithium and treated in independent depressive episodes with NTP had full responses to this last antidepressant. On the other hand, the AMI and CMI biotransformation may also be central in some of the apparent discrepancies encountered in the prediction studies for TADs responses using different indices of monoaminergic turnover (10,21,22).

Finally, it must be emphasized that the existence of a probable interdependence between TADs and lithium effectiveness could contribute to better understanding of the biological correlates of MAD. In fact, this finding may reasonably be considered to prove that NTP, DMI and lithium restore and stabilize common abnormalities which are specifically operant in responders to these treatments and are quite different from those involved in the AMI and CMI responders. Therefore searches for similarities and discrepancies in the activities of TADs and lithium at different sites in the brain could help to individuate the key errors that specifically underly the disease in the various meaningful subgroups of patients.

SUICIDAL BEHAVIOR

Proclivity to suicide seems to target a rather specific subgroup of MAD patients with their own neurochemical, pharmacological and possibly genetic-familial patterns (34, 35, 36). Assuming this to be valid, we considered it pertinent to evaluate whether or not suicide-prone MAD patients have, as a group, definite and homogeneous prognoses for long term lithium prophylaxis (37).

Retrospective examination for suicidal behavior before lithium treatment in 49 MAD patients with a mean of 6 depressive breakdowns gave a suicidal rate of 36.8% and showed a high morbidity within the group of suicide attempters, since 43% had histories of multiple suicide attempts.

The two subpopulations of MAD patients so generated, the first with and the second without any apparent proclivity for suicidal acts, had clearly different responses during the subsequent lithium maintenance therapy. Fourteen of 18 patients with histories of suicide attempts were classified as poor lithium responders, while 18 of 31 patients not prone to suicide were good responders (chi square = 5.9; p < .025). The criterion "previous suicidal behavior" as a predictor of a substantial ineffectiveness of lithium maintenance therapy (Table 8) led to 65.3% correct predictions and had a specificity of 78% and a sensitivity of 58%. The high specificity indicates that a positive history of suicidal acts seems to be truly connected with a subsequent poor lithium prognosis, while the lower sensitivity indicates that the reverse relationship, that is no suicides, would be indicative of good lithium responsiveness, is weaker.A lack of suicidal behavior must be utilized cautiously as a predictor for good lithium response.

Table 8. Suicidal behavior and lithium outcome in MAD.

Specificity	78%	False positives	8.2%
Sensitivity	58%	False negatives	26.5%
	Correct prediction	65.3%	

The higher concentration of poor lithium responders among suicide-prone patients is not easily referred to a more violent form of disease within this group: in fact, prior to beginning long term lithium, suicide attempters had similar rates per year of affective episodes and, in the various key episodes, similar depression scores as patients without any history of self-destructive acts. On the other hand, the observation that 6 of 9 probands on lithium and without personal histories of suicide attempts but with suicide victims among first degree relatives had poor lithium prognosis strengthens the hypothesis that poor lithium responders might actually have some internal characteristics, intimately connected and apparently running in familly, along with being prone to suicidal behavior.

Data indicating lower 5HIAA accumulation in the CSF of MAD patients appears always to be associated with higher chance of suicidal behavior, with a frequency near that of failure in long term lithium prophylaxis (38), together with evidence that chiefly high MHPG excre-

tors - who are the patients most likely to have concomit-
antly lower 5HT turnover(10) - are candidates for a poor
lithium outcome (26), contribute independently to linking
both poor lithium response and increased risk for suicide
to lowered 5HT turnover and to support indirectly the
finding that being prone to suicide may be a real predictor for poor lithium outcome.

CONCLUSIONS

The data presented undoubtedly suggest that each of
the selected variables offers possibilities for prediction
of the effectiveness of long term lithium prophylaxis:
correct selections ranged between 95.7% and 58.7%, with
fluctations in specificity from 100% to 68% and in sensitivity from 100% to 50%.

However these results must be at this time considered
only to express relationships which are pertinent to
the particular sample being analyzed and generalizations
must be evoided. The relatively limited size of the sample
of patients prevents us from concluding that we are in
truth dealing with true predictors and emphasizes the
high priority for supplementary investigation. It is
also obvious that at least for some variables, especially
the urinary MHPG in bipolars and the response to DMI,
the specificities and sensitivities estimated are too
optimistic and more representative samples will lead
in the future to lower predictive powers. It must be
finally taken into account that while we have selected
patients with a severe form of disease and with substantially all-or-nothing lithium responses, in clinical
practice   milder cases for whom the evaluation of the
effectiveness of lithium prophylaxis may be more ambiguous

are often given lithium. Therefore, our data are attractive and promising for both the clinical and the research
fields but should not be used as yet for decisions about
long term lithium treatment.

We are convinced that our results cannot be simply
referred to chance, since the weight of the associations
between each of the tested variables and the different
lithium outcomes is straightforward.
Therefore we will focus in more detail on the specific
issue of the inherent characteristics of the predictors
and of the possibilities of further development of improved procedures of prediction.

For the item "inherent characteristics of the prediction", an analysis of those factors which may have played
limiting roles in our observations is particularly important.

Misclassification can be due, in theory, not only
to factors specific for variables tested from time to
time as possible predictors and which have been briefly
 summarized when commenting on the specific results,
but also to three main general sources of errors.

The first source of error is that the number of individuals who meet or do not meet a definite selection criterion may differ importantly from the numbers of suc-
cessful or unsuccessful responders to lithium: working
with "rare" predictors, sensitivity is lost, while working with "overrepresented" predictors, the specificity
falls because of an inevitable increase in the number
of false positives.

The second source of error is that there is unlikely
a simple unifactorial foundation for differences in lithium effectiveness. In this context, a relative excess

of false positives would indicate that the criterion of selection is a phenotypic expression of some peculiarity of primary importance in influencing the predicted lithium response, even though for its full manifestation the concomitance of other factors is required. On the contrary, an elevated frequency of false negatives would suggest that the criterion of selection expresses some factor playing a more accessory, permissive role in determining long term lithium effectiveness.

The third source of error is that we are in any case dealing with indirect indices that express only more or less partially those underlying abnormalities that are per se responsible for different lithium outcomes.

For all these reasons, it is clear that easy formulations based on single effects cannot be utilized to obtain correct explanations for both false positives and false negatives. It is, however, equally clear that attempts to precisely weigh the direct and indirecting powers of the different possible sources of error is arduous, since some of them are not really quantifiable. Therefore, it is easy to predict that at best some remaining fraction of misclassification will be unexplained, even when methodologically sophisticated strategies will have been applied.

As it is, with regard to the item "prospects of developing improved procedures of selections", it must be stressed that the need for this could be at least partially bypassed by reducing the operational consequences of the erratic information included in each predictor. In fact, the error of classification due to false positives or to false negatives weighs differently for different investigational purposes, with specificity being more important sometime and sensitivity others. Therefore proper choice of selection criteria may serve as a buffer against misclassification; in spite of this possibility of internally compensating for the errors, however, it would be useful to acquire selection procedures with better specificity and sensitivity. There are two strategies for doing this, one centered on a search for new and more precise predictors and the other based on combining previously acquired predictors. The first trend will undoubtedly be helpful to obtain more precise information about the mechanisms underlying the disease in patients who are responsive or unresponsive to lithium. It is probably less useful if specifically aimed at fully satisfactorily grouping patients according to their own future prognosis with lithium. Because of the obviously multifactorial nature of the processes that affect the heterogeneity of lithium responses, the search for a unique variable that can justify nearly all the variance is probably a waste of time.

It should be more useful to obtain better prediction by combining multiple putative predictors of lithium outcome. In this way, each patient would be described by a cumulative value indicative of all the different variables and, along the continuum of values so obtained, a theoretical threshold for separating out a quote of misclassifications, with single predictors should appear.

This procedure, which requires the application to large numbers of patients of mathematical models such as stepwise, multivariate or cluster analyses, is undoubtedly laborious, but its potentially rewarding prospects indicate that it would be worthwhile to proceed in this direction.

REFERENCES

1. Prien, R. F. (1979). Clinical use of lithium - Part I: Introduction. In: Cooper, T.B., Gershon, S., Kline, N.S. and Schou, M. (eds). Lithium: Controversies and Unresolved Issues. pp. 3-29. (Amsterdam: Excerpta Medica)

2. Georgotas, A. and Gershon, S. (1979). Lithium in manic-depressive illness: some highlights and current controversies. In: Cooper, T.B., Gershon, S., Kline, N.S. and Schou, M. (eds). Lithium: Controversies and Unresolved Issues. pp. 57-84. (Amsterdam: Excerpta Medica)

3. Gerbino, L., Oleshansky, M. and Gershon, S. (1978). Clinical use and mode of action of lithium. In: Lipton, M.A., Di Mascio, A. and Killam, K.F. (eds). Psychopharmacology: A Generation of Progress. pp. 1261-75. (New York: Raven Press)

4. Carrol, B.J. (1979). Prediction of treatment outcome with lithium. In: Cooper, T.B., Gershon, S., Kline, N.S. and Schou, M. (eds). Lithium: Controversie and Unresolved Issues. pp. 171-97. (Amsterdam: Excerpta Medica)

5. Frazer, A., Mendels, J., Ramsky, T.A. et al. (1979). Erythrocyte concentrations of the lithium ion. In: Cooper, T.B., Gershon, S., Kline, N.S. and Schou, M. (eds). Lithium: Controversies and Unresolved Issues. pp. 198-208. (Amsterdam: Excerpta Medica)

6. Cazzullo, C.L., Sacchetti, E. and Smeraldi, E. (1979). Psychotropic drugs and their relationship with psychopatology of affective disorders. Progress in Neuropsychopharmacol., 3, 25-38

7. Cazzullo, C.L., Sacchetti, E. and Smeraldi, E. New trends on long term lithium treatment in affective disorders. In: Cazzullo, C.L. and Invernizzi, G. (eds). Prevention in Psychiatry. (1979) . pp. 115-30. (Milano: Edi Ermes)

8. Emrich, H.M. (1982). Prophylactic therapies in affective disorders: mode of action from a clinical point of view. In: Emrich, H.M., Aldenhoff, J.B. and Lux, H.D. (eds). Basic Mechanisms in the Action of Lithium. pp. 202-14. (Amsterdam: Excerpta Medica)

9. Post, R.M. and Goodwin, F.K. (1978). Approaches to brain amines in psychiatric patients: a reevaluation of cerebrospinal fluid studies. In: Iversen, L.L., Iversen S.D. and Snyder, S.H. (eds). Handbook of Psychopharmacology. Biology of Mood and Antianxiety Drugs. pp. 147-85. (New York: Plenum Press)

10. Goodwin, F.K., Cowdry, R.W. and Webster M.H. (1978). Predictors of drug response in the affective disorders:

towards an integrated approach. In: Lipton, M.A., Di Mascio A. and Killam, K.F. (eds). Psychopharmacology: A Generation of Progress. pp. 1277-88. (New York: Raven Press)

11. van Praag, H.M. (1978). Amine hypothesis of affective disorders. In: Iversen, L.L., Iversen, S.D. and Snyder, S.H. (eds). Handbook of Psychopharmacology. Biology of Mood and Antianxiety Drugs. pp. 187-297. (New York: Plenum Press)

12. Sacchetti, E. and Smeraldi, E. (1980). MHPG e depressione primaria: una rivalutazione delle ipotesi monoaminergiche tradizionali. In: Smeraldi, E. and Sacchetti, E. (eds). La Depressione come Problema Psicobiologico. pp. 49-79. (Milano: Edi Ermes)

13. Schatzberg, A.F., Orsulak, P.J., Rosenbaum, A.H. et al. (1983). Biochemical subtypes of unipolar depressives. In: Clayton, P.J. and Barret, J.E. (eds). Treatment of Depression: Old Controversies and New Approaches. pp. 53-9. (New York: Raven Press)

14. Winokur, G. (1978). Mania and depression: family studies and genetics in relation to treatment. In: Lipton, M.A., Di Mascio, A. and Killam, K.F. (eds). Psychopharmacology: A Generation of Progress. pp. 1213-21. (New York: Raven Press)

15. Maas, J.W. (ed) (1983). MHPG: Basic Mechanisms and Psychopatology. (New York: Academic Press)

16. Cazzullo, C.L., Smeraldi, E., Sacchetti, E. and Bottinelli, S. (1975). Intracellular lithium concentration and clinical response. Brit. J. Psychiat., 126, 298-300

17. Sacchetti, E., Bottinelli, S., Bellodi, L. et al. (1977). Erythrocyte/plasma lithium ratios. Lancet, i, 908

18. Feighner, J.P., Robins, E., Guze, S. et al. (1972). Diagnostic criteria for use in psychiatric research. Arch. Gen. Psychiatry., 26, 57-63

19. American Psychiatric Association, Committee on nomenclature and statistics: Diagnostic and Statistical Manual of Mental Disorders, ed. III. (1980) (Washington D.C.: A.P.A.)

20. Cazzullo, C.L. and Sacchetti, E. Critical issues in the evaluation of long term lithium treatment. In this volume.

21. Cazzullo, C.L., Sacchetti, E., Allaria, E. et al. (1982). Is urinary MHPG a real predictor of drug response in Primary Depression? In: Costa, E. and Racagni, G. (eds). Typical and Atypical Antidepressants: Clinical Practice. pp. 237-47. (New York: Raven Press)

22. Beckmann, H. and Goodwin, F.K. (1980). Urinary MHPG

in subgroups of depressed patients and normal controls. Neuropsychobiology., 6, 91-100

23. Sacchetti, E., Allaria, E., Negri, F. et al. (1979). 3-methoxy-4-hydroxyphenylglycol and primary depression: clinical and pharmacological considerations. Biol. Psychiatry., 14, 473-84

24. Maas, J.K. (1978). Clinical implications of pharmacological differences among antidepressants. In: Lipton, M.A., Di Mascio, A. and Killam, K.F. (eds). Psychopharmacology: A Generation of Progress. pp. 955-60. (New York: Raven Press)

25. Maas, J.W., Kocsic, J.H., Bowden, C.L. et al. (1982) Pre-treatment neurotransmitter metabolites and response to imipramine or amitriptyline treatment. Psychological Medicine., 12, 37-43

26. Sacchetti, E., Faravelli, C., Conte, G. et al. Monoaminergic profiles in major affective disorders and clinical response to long term lithium treatment. A four-to-six years follow up. Submitted for publication.

27. Angst, J. and Grof, P. (1979). Selection of patients with recurrent affective illness for a long term study: testing research criteria on prospective follow up data. In: Cooper, T.B., Geshon, S., Kline, N.S. and Schou, M. (eds). Lithium: Controversies and Unresolved Issues. pp. 355-69. (Amsterdam: Excerpta Medica)

28. Zis, A.P., Grof., P. and Goodwin, F.K. (1979). The natural course of affective disorders: implications for lithium prophylaxis. In: Cooper, T.B., Gershon, S., Kline, N.S. and Schou, M. (eds). Lithium: Controversie and Unresolved Issues. pp. 381-98. (Amsterdam: Excerpta Medica)

29. Omenn, G.S. and Motulsky, A.G. (1975). Pharmacogenetics: clinical and experimental studies in man. In: Eleftheriou, B.E. (ed). Psychopharmacogenetics. pp. 183-228. (New York: Plenum Press)

30. Faravelli, C., Broadhurst, A., James, H. and Sacchetti, E. (1981). Pharmacokinetic, clinical and biological parameters modulating the response to chlorimipramine. In: Perris, C., Struwe, G. and Jansson, B. (eds). Biological Psychiatry 1981. pp. 1167-70. (Amsterdam: Elsevier/North Holland Biomedical Press)

31. Sacchetti, E. Depressione primaria: ruolo dell'eterogeneità biochimica nella modulazione dell'effetto terapeutico dei sali di litio e dei farmaci antidepressivi. Proceedings of the XXXV Congress of the Italian Society of Psychiatry. In press

32. Sacchetti, E., Vita, A., Conte, G. et al.   Long

term lithium effectiveness in major affective disorders: relationship to tricyclic antidepressants responsiveness. In preparation

33. Buchsbaum, M.S., Maier, R.J. and Murphy, D.L. (1977) Suicide attempts, platelet monoamine oxidase and the average evoked response. Acta Psychiat. Scand., 56, 69-79

34. Brown, G.L., Goodwin, F.K. and Bunney, W.E. Jr. (1982). Human aggression and suicide: their relationship to neuropsychiatric diagnoses and serotonin metabolism. In: Ho, B.T., Schoolar, J.C. and Usdin, E. (eds). Serotonin in Biological Psychiatry. pp. 287-307. (New York: Raven Press)

35. Traskman, L., Åsberg, M., Bertilsson, L. and Sjostrand, L. (1981). Monoamine metabolites in CSF and suicidal behavior. Arch. Gen. Psychiatry., 38, 831-36

36. Montgomery, S.A. and Montgomery, D.B. (1982). Drug treatment of suicidal behavior. In: Costa, E. and Racagni, G. (eds). Typical and Atypical Antidepressants: Clinical Practice. pp. 347-55. (New York: Raven Press)

37. Sacchetti, E., Conte, G., Vita, A. et al. Proneness to suicidal behavior in major depressives identifies homogeneous pharmacological patterns. In preparation

38. van Praag, H.M. (1982). Serotonin precursors in the treatment of depression. In: Ho, B.T., Schoolar, J.C. and Usdin, E. (eds). Serotonin in Biological Psychiatry. pp. 259-86. (New York: Raven Press)

Supported by CNR Contract N° 82.02298.56 to Dr. E. Sacchetti.

14
Practical value of biological and phByschological indicators in predicting response to lithium prophylaxis of manic-depressive psychosis

M. MAJ, F. ARENA, R. PIROZZI AND D. KEMALI

INTRODUCTION

The role of lithium as an effective agent in preventing recurrence of manic-depressive psychosis is now well established. It has been repeatedly reported, however, that about 20 to 50% of manic-depressive patients relapse over a two-year period during lithium prophylaxis. Since this treatment involves the risk of adverse reactions (mainly, impairment of renal concentrating ability), it would be desirable to rely on effective predictors of response, which allow to prescribe lithium selectively to patients who are likely to benefit from it. By the other hand, since manic-depressive psychosis is thought to be a heterogeneous condition from a biological point of view, the identification of specific features of lithium responsive and non-responsive patients would be also of theoretical interest, bringing to further understanding of the pathophysiology of the illness.

A variety of potential predictors of response to prophylactic lithium have been proposed in the past years. Among clinical variables, a definite diagnosis of bipolar affective illness (1) and a family history of bipolar affective disorders (2) have been regarded as indicators of a good response, whereas rapid cycling (i.e., the occurrence of more than three affective episodes within one year) (3), a

history of alcoholism or drug abuse not associated with mood changes
(4), and the presence of paranoid features in the clinical picture (4)
have been cited as predictors of a poor outcome. On the biological side, a high red blood cell/plasma lithium ratio (5) and a significantly
elevated potential difference across the rectal mucosa (6) have been
found to be associated with a favourable response to prophylaxis, while the presence of the HLA-A3 antigen has been reported to be significantly more frequent in non-responsive patients (7,8). Finally, psychological studies have claimed evidence of higher mean scores on the
Obsessional Scale of the Middlesex Hospital Questionnaire in lithium-
responsive patients (9) and on the Neuroticism Scale of the Eysenck
Personality Questionnaire in non-responders (10).

Most of the above mentioned studies have been concerned with only
one or few potential predictors, and have reported a large overlap
between responders and non-responders with regard to the examined variable thus limiting its practical significance as a real "predictor"
of response. Moreover, some of these investigations appear to be cri-
ticizable from a methodological point of view: prophylactic periods
are sometimes too short (less than one year), or different from one
patient to another (which is incorrect, since the likelihood of recurrences rises with time) or not compared with identical pre-lithium periods (so that evaluation of response is not reliable).

In the present investigation, we have tested the predictive value
of several socio-demographic, clinical, biological, and psychological
variables, extending prophylactic period to two years, and selecting
for the study only patients who had suffered from at least two affective episodes within the two years before starting lithium treatment.
SUBJECTS AND METHODS
100 patients (40 males and 60 females, age range 25-70 yrs., mean $\pm$
SD 46.5 $\pm$ 10.7) were admitted to the study. Inclusion criteria were a
diagnosis of bipolar affective psychosis or unipolar depressive psychosis according to Perris (11) and a history of at least two affective

episodes within the two years preceding the start of lithium treatment.
51 patients were diagnosed as bipolars and 49 as unipolars. All patients were treated for two years with lithium carbonate, conventional
form, at doses ranging from 600 to 1500 mg/day, and maintained at plasma lithium levels of 0.6-1.0 mEq/l. They were visited monthly or by-
monthly. Psychopathological state was assessed by CPRS (12) and Hamilton Rating Scale for Depression (13). We classified as "non-responders"
to prophylaxis those patients (no.=41) who had one or more relapses
during the two-year follow-up period, requiring hospitalization and/or
treatment with significant doses of specific drugs (antidepressants or
neuroleptics), and as "responders" those patients (no.=59) who did not
relapse during the follow-up period.

The socio-demographic variables recorded in each patient were: 1)
sex, 2) age at the start of lithium treatment, 3)marital status, 4)so-
cial class (according to Hollingshead and Redlich, 14), 5)years of
schooling, 6) major problem areas at the start of lithium treatment
(checked by a semi-structured interview). The clinical and historical
variables explored, by interviewing the patient and all available relatives, were: 1)type of affective illness (if bipolar or unipolar),
2) age at the onset of the illness, 3) duration of the illness, 4) number of episodes per year, 5)family history of affective psychoses,
6)family history of bipolar affective psychosis.

During lithium prophylaxis each patient was administered, while
being euthymic, the Middlesex Hospital Questionnaire (15) and the
Eysenck Personality Questionnaire (16).

Biological investigation included determination of: 1) plasma lithium concentration (on the occasion of each visit, by flame photometry) 2) red blood cell/plasma lithium ratio (at least twice during the
follow-up period, by atomic absorption spectrophotometry, as described
in 17), 3) platelet MAO activity (at least twice during the follow-up
period, testing each patient while being euthymic, by a radioenzymatic
method using tryptamine and beta-phenylethylamine as substrates, as

Table I.   Socio-demographic variables and response to prophylactic
          lithium

Variable	Responders(n=59)	Non-responders(n=41)
SEX		
Male	21 (52.5%)	19 (47.5%)
Female	38 (63.3%)	22 (36.7%)
AGE AT THE START OF LITHIUM		
17-40 years	27 (65.8%)	14 (34.2%)
41-60 years	29 (53.7%)	25 (46.3%)
More than 60 years	3 (60.0%)	2 (40.0%)
MARITAL STATUS		
Married	42 (60.9%)	27 (39.1%)
Single,separated,divorced		
or widoved	17 (54.8%)	14 (45.2%)
SOCIAL CLASS^		
I-II	7 (58.3%)	5 (41.7%)
III	38 (62.3%)	23 (37.7%)
IV	10 (55.5%)	8 (44.5%)
V	4 (44.4%)	5 (55.6%)
YEARS OF SCHOOLING		
0-8	31 (62.0%)	19 (38.0%)
9-13	16 (59.2%)	11 (40.8%)
14 or more	12 (52.2%)	11 (47.8%)
MAJOR PROBLEM AREAS AT THE START		
OF LITHIUM		
Marital/Familial	20 (57.1%)	15 (42.9%)
Work/Financial	3 (30.0%)	7 (70.0%)
Social/Interpersonal	4 (66.7%)	2 (33.3%)
None	32 (65.3%)	17 (34.7%)

^According to Hollingshead and Redlich (14)

described in 18), and 4) HLA antigens (by the standard NIH microcytoto-
xicity test, as detailed in 8).

Statistical significance of differences between responders and non-
responders was evaluated by the Student's t test and the χ^2 method with
Yates' correction. Moreover, a stepwise discriminant analysis between
the two patient groups was performed, according to the program of Jen-
nrich and Sampson (19).

RESULTS

No significant relationship was found between socio-demographic variables and response to lithium prophylaxis (table I).

Among clinical and historical variables (table II), a positive family history of bipolar affective illness resulted to be significantly
more frequent ($p < 0.05$) in lithium-responsive patients than in non-responders. A higher response rate was found in bipolars as compared
with unipolars, but the difference was not significant. A non-signi-
cant trend of patients with a history of more than two affective episodes per year to be refractory to prophylaxis was noticed.

Non-responders showed higher mean scores than responders on each of
the subscales of Middlesex Hospital Questionnaire (table III), but
none of the differences reached a significant level. Mean score on the
Neuroticism Scale of the Eysenck Personality Questionnaire was significantly higher ($p < 0.01$) in non-responders, whereas a non-significant
trend of responders to show higher extraversion scores was recorded.

Mean values of lithium ratio were significantly higher ($p < 0.01$)
in responders than in non-responders (table IV), whereas no significant
difference between the two groups was found with respect to plasma lithium concentration and platelet MAO activity. The frequency of the
HLA-A3 antigen was found to be significantly higher($p < 0.01$) in the
group of non-responders(table V).

On stepwise discriminant analysis, as a F-to-enter of 4.000 was
adopted, three variables (score on the Neuroticism Scale of Eysenck
Questionnaire, lithium ratio and HLA-A3 antigen) entered into the clas-

Table II. Clinical/historical variables and response to prophylactic
          lithium

Variable	Responders(n=59)	Non-responders(n=41)
TYPE OF AFFECTIVE ILLNESS		
Bipolar	32 (62.7%)	19 (37.3%)
Unipolar	27 (55.1%)	22 (44.9%)
AGE AT ONSET (yrs.,mean $\pm$ SD)	29.8 $\pm$ 8.4	32.7 $\pm$ 10.5
DURATION OF ILLNESS		
(yrs.,mean $\pm$ SD)	12.1 $\pm$ 8.6	12.0 $\pm$ 10.0
NUMBER OF EPISODES PER YEAR		
Less than 1.0	28 (63.6%)	16 (36.4%)
1.0-2.0	28 (59.6%)	19 (40.4%)
More than 2.0	3 (33.3%)	6 (66.7%)
FAMILY HISTORY OF AFFECTIVE PSYCHOSES		
Positive	25 (73.5%)	9 (26.5%)
Negative	34 (51.5%)	32 (48.5%)
FAMILY HISTORY OF BIPOLAR AFFECTIVE PSYCHOSIS		
Positive	19 (82.6%)^	4 (17.4%)
Negative	40 (51.9%)	37 (48.1%)

^$p < 0.05$

sification functions. Jackknifed classification matrix showed that these functions classified correctly 74.6% of responders and 68.3% of non-
responders (table VI).

DISCUSSION

The results of our investigation confirm the potential role as predictors of response to lithium prophylaxis of four indices: a positive family history of bipolar affective illness and a high lithium ratio (po-

Table III. Psychological variables and response to prophylactic lithium

Variable	Responders(n=59)	Non-responders(n=41)
SCORES ON THE SCALES OF MIDDLESEX HOSPITAL QUESTIONNAIRE (mean $\pm$ SD)		
Anxiety	6.47 ± 2.70	7.20 ± 2.70
Phobic	4.38 ± 2.54	5.00 ± 1.67
Obsessional	6.19 ± 2.76	6.50 ± 3.57
Somatic	3.41 ± 2.40	3.42 ± 1.95
Depression	4.92 ± 3.95	4.95 ± 1.80
Hysteria	2.69 ± 2.30	3.10 ± 2.90
SCORES ON THE SCALES OF EYSENCK PERSONALITY QUESTIONNAIRE (mean $\pm$ SD)		
Psychoticism	3.25 ± 1.85	3.80 ± 1.64
Extraversion	11.70 ± 5.30	10.25 ± 6.09
Neuroticism	9.34 ± 3.80	11.95 ± 4.28^

^$p < 0.01$

sitive indicators) and the presence of the HLA-A3 antigen and a high score on the Neuroticism Scale of Eysenck Questionnaire (negative indicators).

A large overlap between responders and non-responders with regard to each of these variables was observed. Nevertheless, neuroticism score lithium ratio and HLA-A3 antigen, considered together, classified correctly 72.0% of patients. Therefore, it seems that, although none of these variables can predict prophylaxis outcome by itself, they might have a real predictive value if taken as a group.

On the basis of the reported findings, it can be hypothesized that

Table IV. BIOCHEMICAL/PHARMACOKINETIC VARIABLES AND RESPONSE TO PROPHY-
         LACTIC LITHIUM

Variable	Responders(n=59)	Non-responders(n=41)
MEAN PLASMA LITHIUM CONCENTRA-TION (mEq/l)	0.65 ± 0.07	0.66 ± 0.08
MEAN RBC/PLASMA LITHIUM RATIO	0.40 ± 0.08^	0.36 ± 0.05
MEAN PLATELET MAO ACTIVITY (tryptamine, nmoles/mg prot./hr)	5.55 ± 1.60	5.48 ± 1.72
MEAN PLATELET MAO ACTIVITY (beta-phenylethylamine, nmoles/ mg prot./hr)	12.30 ± 3.29	12.20 ± 3.16

All values expressed as mean $\pm$ SD

^$p < 0.01$

a significant role in the failure of lithium prophylaxis may be played by pharmacogenetic factors, i.e., an impaired transport of the
lithium ion into the cells, probably as an effect of peculiar cell
membrane characteristics (presence of specific HLA antigens). It must
be mentioned, in this connection, that the presence of HLA-A3 antigen
was found to be significantly more frequent, within our sample, in
patients with lithium ratio values below the median as compared with
those whose values were above the median, thus confirming data previously reported by our group (8).

   As regards the association between high scores on the Neuroticism
Scale of the Eysenck Questionnaire and poor response to lithium, it
can be perhaps postulated that when neurotic traits are present in
the patient's personality lithium treatment is not sufficient to
prevent relapses, and an associated psychoterapeutic approach is
needed. Further studies on large populations of patients are, however, required to settle this issue adequately.

Table V. HLA ANTIGENS AND RESPONSE TO PROPHYLACTIC LITHIUM

HLA ANTIGEN	% DISTRIBUTION	
	Responders (n=59)	Non-responders (n=41)
A1	18.6	12.2
A2	38.9	48.8
A3	15.2	41.5^
A9	27.1	12.2
A10	16.9	17.1
A11	22.0	9.8
A28	1.7	7.3
A29	18.6	9.8
B5	11.9	14.6
B7	18.6	12.2
B8	5.1	4.9
B12	15.2	9.8
B13	8.5	7.3
B14	3.4	12.2
B15	10.2	12.2
B17	8.5	9.8
B18	18.6	14.6
Bw21	1.6	0
Bw22	5.1	2.4
B27	0	4.9
Bw35	44.1	36.6
B37	1.7	2.4
B38	3.4	7.3
B39	3.4	0
Bw40	0	2.4
Bw45	5.1	0
Bw49	1.7	0
Cw3	6.8	7.3
Cw4	40.7	41.5

^p<0.01

Table VI. STEPWISE DISCRIMINANT ANALYSIS. JACKKNIFED CLASSIFICATION
MATRIX (FUNCTIONS: NEUROTICISM SCORE ON EPQ, LITHIUM RATIO,
HLA-A3 ANTIGEN)

| GROUP | NO.PATIENTS | NO. CASES CLASSIFIED INTO GROUP | | PERCENT CORRECT |
		RESPONDERS	NON-RESPONDERS	
RESPONDERS	59	44	15	74.6
NON-RESPONDERS	41	13	28	68.3
TOTAL	100	57	43	72.0

REFERENCES

1.Fieve,R.R.,Kumbaraci,T. and Dunner D.L. (1976). Lithium prophylaxis of depression in bipolar I, bipolar II, and unipolar patients.Arch.
Gen.Psychiat.,133,925-929

2.Mendlewicz,J.,Fieve,R.R. and Stallone F. (1973) Relationship between
the effectiveness of lithium therapy and family history.Am.J.Psychiat.
130,1011-1013

3.Dunner,D.L. and Fieve R.R. (1974). Clinical factors in lithium prophylactic failure.Arch.Gen.Psychiat.,30,229-233

4.Prien,R.F. and Caffey,E.M. (1977). Long term maintenance drug therapy
in recurrent affective illness: current status and issues.Dis.Nerv.
Syst.,38,981-992

5.Mendels,J.,Frazer,A.,Baron,J.,Kukopulos,A.,Reginaldi,A.,Tondo,L. and
Cagliari,B. (1976) Intra-erythrocyte lithium ion concentration and
long-term maintenance treatment.Lancet i:966

6.Peet,M. (1975). The potential difference across the rectal mucosa
during depressive illness and lithium therapy.Brit.J.Psychiat.,127,
144-148

7.Perris,C.,Strandman,E. and Wåhlby,L. (1979). HL-A antigens and response to prophylactic lithium.Neuropsychobiol.,5,114-118

8.Del Vecchio,M.,Farzati,B.,Maj,M.,Minucci,P.,Guida,L. and Kemali,D. (1981). Cell membrane predictors of response to lithium prophylaxis of affective disorders.Neuropsychobiol.,7,243-247

9.Kerry,R.J. and Orme,J.E. (1979)Lithium,manic-depressive illness and psychological test performance.Brit.Med.J.,1,230

10.Coppen,A.,Metcalfe,M. and Bailey,J. (1979). Lithium prophylactic therapy in unipolar depression and some possible prognosticators of response. In:Copper,T.B.,Gershon,S.,Kline,N.S. and Schou,M. (eds.). Lithium:controversies and unresolved issues. pp.401-412. (Amsterdam: Excerpta Medica)

11.Perris,C. (1966). A study of bipolar (manic-depressive) and unipolar recurrent depressive psychosis.Acta Psychiat. Scand. Suppl.,194

12.Perris,C.,Kemali,D.,Amati,A.,Del Vecchio,M. and Vacca,L. (1981). CPRS:scala di valutazione psicopatologica globale.Neurol. Psichiat. Sci. Umane,1,232-276

13.Hamilton,M. (1960) A rating scale for depression.J. Neurol. Neuro-surg. Psychiat.,23,56-62

14.Hollingshead,A.B. and Redlich,F.C. (1958)Social class and mental illness.J.Wiley and sons,New York

15.Crown,S. and Crisp,A.H. Manual of the Middlesex Hospital Question-naire (MHQ). Psychological Test Publications, Barstaple

16.Eysenck,H. J. and Eysenck,S.B.G. (1975) Manual of the Eysenck per-sonality questionnaire. Hodder and Stoughton Educational,Kent

17.Del Vecchio,M.,Famiglietti,L.A.,Maj,M.,Zizolfi,S.,Borriello,R. and Sciaudone,G. (1979) Kinetics of lithium and rubidium after a single administration.Acta Neurol. ,34,204-213

18.Del Vecchio,M.,Maj,M.,D'Ambrosio,A. and Kemali,D. (1983) Low platelet MAO activity in chronic schizophrenics:a long-term effect of neuroleptic treatment?.Psychopharmacol.,79,177-179

19.Jennrich,R. and Sampson,P. (1981) Stepwise discriminant analysis.

In:BMPD,Department of Biomathematics,University of California,Los Angeles, pp.519-525

15
Outcome to treatment with lithium in affective patients and family history

E. SMERALDI, F. MACCIARDI, M. GASPERINI AND L. BELLODI

Heterogeneity is one of the main problems in dealing with Affective Disorders and several different approaches have been applied to detect it, but the complex problem of heterogeneity can not be satisfactorily analyzed by symptomatic and/or syndromic strategies. Since the clinical criteria per se seem not to be useful for solving any question, our group designed study to see whether the presence or the absence of response to long-term therapy might differentiate between biologically/biochemically different forms of Affective Disorders. In fact, behind their clinical and phenomenological homogeneity, Affective Disorders may well be etiologically and hence genetically distinct.

In this sense the outcome on Lithium might be a useful criterion for discriminating biological heterogeneity. From a theoretical point of view, we could also use the outcome on tricyclic therapy. However, though anti-depressants act on the biological systems supposed to be related to the origin of affective disease, they are also symptomatic drugs, while the effect of Lithium is rather specific, is the only non-symptomatic treatment in psychiatry and can also be used as a preventive therapy. Patients who do not relapse while on Lithium therapy generally have low MHPG values during their depressive phases and consequently also have good outcomes on tricyclics with noradrenergic profiles (1). Therefore, all that we say about Lithium could also refer to tricyclic pro-noradrenergic antidepressants.

Many controlled studies have established the efficacy of Lithium for the long-term treatment of unipolar and bipolar illness (2). Nevertheless, relapses do occur in some patients. Mendlewicz and his co-workers (3) have hypothesized that genetic factors might account for the heterogeneity of the response. In order to confirm their reports and since we also found a higher frequency of illness in first degree relatives of Lithium non-relapsed subjects (table 1), we submitted our data to a preliminary logistic analysis (4) to see if there are any correlations between the frequency of the illness and some characteristics of the probands and their relatives (table 2). As we can see from this table, the most significant parameter is the mean frequency of the disease among relatives (MR = 13.87% with a Z value of 4.42). The effect of Lithium outcome gives a variation of 8.91% on the mean frequency and the effect of the type of relationship one of 6.04%.

These results show that the frequency of illness is always higher in the relatives of non-relapsed subjects both in sibs and in parents. Finally, even though we could not find any significant effect of sex, since it appears to be linked to a second order interaction of sex of the proband to sex of the relative to the type of relationship,

Table 1. Age-corrected frequency of the affective disorders
in the relatives of relapsed and non-relapsed
probands

	Relapsed probands	Non-relapsed probands
Brothers observed risk %	19.11	44.89
Sisters observed risk %	20.99	39.95
Fathers observed risk %	9.11	28.31
Mothers observed risk %	24.10	20.08

Reproduced from (4).

Table 2. Logistic analysis of main effects

Mean frequency of the disease	$a = 13.87$ %
Lithium outcome	relapsed = $a - 5.55$ %
	non-relapsed = $a + 3.36$ %
Type of relationship	parents = $a - 3.23$ %
	siblings = $a + 2.81$ %

Reproduced from (4).

which is not easily detectable with the analysis utilized,
we feel that is more correct and useful to take into
account a trend of sex and therefore we used models which
also consider differences in sex.

Our data suggest that there are some links between the
genetic mechanisms that underly the Affective Disorders and

those that underly the response to Lithium, but from a strictly genetic point of view there are some limitations, mainly because we have not gathered in past studies any information about the number of families and the size of each family investigated.

There are now genetic methods that can include this information, and therefore, we have now analyzed the frequency of illness in the relatives of a group of patients with Affective Disorders treated for long time with Lithium. We then applied a computational genetic model including a sex effect (5) to our data, with reclassification of our probands as relapsed or non-relapsed (6), to avoid the responder/non-responder dichotomy, since this dichotomy would need to testing to establish a direct link between the pharmacological effects of Lithium and the biological structure of the proband.

This type of analysis does not enable us to rule out either the Single Major Locus (SML) nor the Multifactorial Polygenic (MFP) hypothesis of transmission, but some specific trends of the two groups have been elicited. We found a sex effect (women are more affected than men) for the group of relapsed patients and low values of penetrance in heterozygotes with a trend toward recessivity with the SML. On the contrary, the parametric set of the SML model for the group of non-relapsed patients shows a pattern of dominance and a reduced sex effect. All this suggest that the group of non-relapsed consists of more homogeneous subjects from the clinical and genetic points of view. The MFP model further confirms this hypothesis, since for the group of non-relapsed there was no sex effect but the sibling and parent-offspring correlations were higher than for the relapsed group.

The estimated values for the illness allele q for the
two models are very different. The reliability of these
results is indirectly proven by the results of the analysis
of the expected frequencies of the disease in the general
population generated by the models, which gives a total
value of 5.6 %, a value reliable for the Italian population (Table 3) (7, 8).

Table 3. Morbidity Risk for Affective Disorders in general
population

	International Data*	Institute of Clinical Psychiatry of Milan**
Bipolar Disorder	0.3 % – 0.88 %	0.56 %
Non Bipolar Disorders	0.6 % – 12 %	7.4 %
	(3% males,4.9% females)	(3.1% males,4.3% females)

* (7)
** (8)

These findings are suggestive but not really conclusive
because in multiple threshold models, since they deal with
disease rates in the group of first degree relatives,
information related to segregation in each family becomes
lost and consequently the solutions obtained do not differ
as much from each other as would be expected in genetic
analysis, because they are mean values for each group.
Nevertheless, more precise investigation utilizing
segregation analysis for single families is now possible
and this provides greater accuracy since it enables us to
enlarge the experimental information to include the second

degree relatives, without losing any information related to the pharmacological heterogeneity. The segregation model we applied (9) is the LIPED (10) , which estimates the Likelihood for each family tested against any specific parametric hypothetical set we choose to describe the susceptibility locus for the disease. At present we have two parametric sets that correspond to two different alternative genetic hypotheses for the identification of the susceptibility locus: we tested the segregation pattern for every family twice, that is for each family we assumed in turn the two different sets of parameters, the first related to the SML genetic structure of the non-relapsed probands and the second to that of relapsed. For each family we obtained two Likelihood values and we were able to calculate the ratio of the two Likelihoods.

This ratio is an index of how well a family fits one or another of the models proposed.

In Table 4 are listed the ratios for those families who segregate better according to the dominant SML model of Lithium non-relapsed probands.

There is a quite random distribution of polarity with 9 Unipolar (UP) and 15 Bipolar (BP).

There is good but not absolute agreement between the genetic system and the clinical pharmacological characteristic of the lithium outcome, since there are 5 families in 24 whose probands relapsed. We do not really have exhaustive information about natural history of our probands' disease. These patients might also have had a good responste to lithium treatment, since lithium therapy might have influenced the rate of recurrence of their episodes of illness.

In Table 5 are the negative likelihood ratios: the

Table 4. Positive Log-Likelihood Ratio Values for Families
of Lithium Treated Affective Probands

Families	Polarity	Clinical Outcome	Ratio
R.E.	Bipolar	Relapsed	2.50
F.L.	Unipolar	Non Relapsed	2.48
B.L.	Bipolar	Non Relapsed	1.28
R.L.	Bipolar	Non Relapsed	1.24
L.G.	Unipolar	Non Relapsed	1.16
O.S.	Bipolar	Non Relapsed	1.06
P.R.	Unipolar	Non Relapsed	1.01
R.N.	Bipolar	Relapsed	0.79
P.A.M.	Unipolar	Non Relapsed	0.58
A.R.	Bipolar	Non Relapsed	0.52
B.A.	Bipolar	Non Relapsed	0.52
Z.E.	Bipolar	Relapsed	0.51
O.P.	Bipolar	Non Relapsed	0.49
R.O.	Unipolar	Relapsed	0.47
S.A.	Bipolar	Non Relapsed	0.42
Al.R.	Bipolar	Non Relapsed	0.32
S.G.L.	Unipolar	Non Relapsed	0.25
B.S.	Bipolar	Non Relapsed	0.25
B.F.	Unipolar	Non Relapsed	0.25
D.F.G.F.	Bipolar	Non Relapsed	0.25
V.A.	Unipolar	Relapsed	0.23
C.L.	Unipolar	Non Relapsed	0.22
G.A.	Bipolar	Non Relapsed	0.20
F.S.	Bipolar	Non Relapsed	0.14

Reproduced from (9)

pattern is quite similar, but a little more complex,
perhaps because of a lesser degree of homogeneity in this
group.

In conclusion, we were trying to test the reliability
of one classification criterion, Lithium outcome, by the
rationale and the methods of formal genetics.

Table 5. Negative Log-Likelihood Ratio Values for Families
of Lithium Treated Affective Probands

Families	Polarity	Clinical Outcome	Ratio
Mo.G.	Unipolar	Non Relapsed	1.26
T.A.	Unipolar	Relapsed	1.26
Bl.A.	Bipolar	Non Relapsed	1.29
Mar.G.	Unipolar	Non Relapsed	1.37
B.C.	Bipolar	Non Relapsed	1.40
P.F.	Bipolar	Non Relapsed	1.41
S.N.	Unipolar	Relapsed	1.41
L.T.	Unipolar	Relapsed	1.43
P.C.	Bipolar	Relapsed	1.50
R.L.	Bipolar	Relapsed	1.50
T.V.	Unipolar	Non Relapsed	1.50
D.R.	Unipolar	Non Relapsed	1.51
G.E.	Unipolar	Non Relapsed	1.53
O.C.	Unipolar	Non Relapsed	1.57
Ca.G.	Bipolar	Relapsed	1.62
D.A.C.	Bipolar	Relapsed	1.65
C.G.	Bipolar	Non Relapsed	1.65
G.F.	Bipolar	Non Relapsed	1.66
Ba.S.	Unipolar	Non Relapsed	1.76
M.I.	Bipolar	Relapsed	1.77
Mag.G.	Bipolar	Non Relapsed	1.85
F.R.	Bipolar	Non Relapsed	1.86
L.M.A.	Bipolar	Non Relapsed	2.00
B.G.	Bipolar	Non Relapsed	2.01
L.E.	Unipolar	Relapsed	2.02
F.M.	Unipolar	Non Relapsed	2.03
P.M.	Bipolar	Relapsed	2.05
T.C.	Bipolar	Relapsed	2.14
Z.P.	Bipolar	Relapsed	2.30
O.S.	Unipolar	Non Relapsed	2.44
C.M.	Bipolar	Non Relapsed	2.57
Zu.G.	Bipolar	Relapsed	2.70
B.E.	Bipolar	Non Relapsed	2.90

Reproduced from (9)

REFERENCES

1. Sacchetti, E. (1983). Lithium prophylaxis in major
affective disorders: on the specificity and sensitivity of
some "new" predictors of treatment outcome. International
meeting on lithium and rubidium therapy . Venice, 30th
september - 2nd october.

2. Cazzullo, C.L., Smeraldi, E. and Sacchetti, E. (1979).
Psychotropic drugs and their relationship with psychopathology of affective disorders. Progr. Neuro-psychopharmacol.,
3, 25-28.

3. Mendlewicz, J. and Stallone, F. (1975). In: Mendlewicz
J. (ed). Genetics and Psychopharmacology. pp. 23-29.
(Basel: Karger).

4. Morabito, A., Gasperini, M., Macciardi, F. and Smeral-
di, E. (1982). Possible relationship between outcome in
Primary Affective Disorders treated with lithium and family
history. In: Costa, E. and Racagni, G. (eds). Typical and
Atypical Antidepressants. pp. 157-163 (New York: Raven
Press).

5. Kidd, K.K. and Spence, M.A. (1976). Genetic analysis
of pyloric stenosis suggesting a specific maternal effect.
J. Med. genet., 13, 290-292.

6. Smeraldi, E., Petroccione, A., Gasperini, M., Macciardi, F., Orsini, A. and Kidd, K.K. . Outcomes on lithium
treatment as a tool for genetic studies in affective disorders. J. Affective Disorders, in press.

7. Boyd, J.H. and Weissman, M.M. (1981). Epidemiology of
affective disorders. A reexamination and future directions.
Arch. Gen. psychiat., 38, 1039-1046.

8. Smeraldi, E., Negri, F., Heimbuch, R.C. and Kidd, K.K.
(1981). Familial patterns and possible models of inheritan
ce of primary affective disorders. J. Affective Disorders,

3, 173–182.

9. Smeraldi, E., Petroccione, A., Gasperini, M., Macciardi, F. and Orsini, A. The search for the genetic homogeneity in affective disorders. Submitted for publication.

10. Morton, L.A. and Kidd, K.K. (1980). The effects of variable age of onset and diagnostic criteria on the estimates of linkage: an example using manic-depressive illness and color blindness. Soc.biol., 27, 1–10.

16
Antidepressant-induced switch and outcome to lithium prophylaxis in bipolar patients

G. CONTE, A. VITA, A. ALCIATI, A. PENNATI AND E. SACCHETTI

One of the most intriguing aspects of the treatment of patients with affective disorders is the drug-induced sudden reversal of mood, from depression to mania or viceversa (1). Bunney reviewed 80 studies involving 3923 patients treated with tricyclic antidepressants or monoamineoxidase inhibitors and found that 9.6 per cent of these patients had switched from depression to mania or hypomania during the treatment (1). Recently it was reported that the frequency of drug-induced switches is much greater in bipolar than in unipolar patients (2).

It has been suggested that susceptibility to induction of mania by a tricyclic antidepressant (TAD) or an MAOi might serve as a biological marker for one subgroup of affectively ill patients (3). On the other hand, a recent work (2) claims that the switch effects of TADs reported in the past probably are random manifestations of bipolar illness, suggesting that a patient may become manic while receiving TADs only by coincidence. To settle this issue, more precise characterization of switch-prone patients in clinical, pharmacological and biological terms seems to be required.

Since homogeneity of response to a specific treatment might be a useful tool for individuating a subgroup of patients with common characteristics (4), one possible way to clarify whether or not switch-prone patients are a meaningful subtype of bipolars would be to test whether or not they react consistently to a particular therapy.

Lithium is generally considered to be the first choice treatment for prophylaxis of recurrence in patients with bipolar affective disorders (5) and is the preminent stabilizing drug against mood swings: therefore we searched the histories of a group of bipolar patients for the occurrence or non-occurrence of drug-induced switches and correlated this with long term outcome to lithium.

SUBJECTS AND METHODS

We retrospectively reviewed the clinical courses of 51 patients selected in accord with the following criteria:
a) they met the DSM 3 criteria for bipolar affective disorder;
b) they had been maintained on lithium therapy for at least 3 years, which is a long enough observation time to clearly indicate the outcome of the treatment for an individual patient; in fact it was demonstrated that during lithium prophylaxis one affective relapse in the first two years of treatment predicted subsequent high rates of recurrences for 78 % of bipolar patients(6).

c) they had had at least five previous episodes since the onset of the disease, with at least two episodes in the last two years before the starting of lithium prophylaxis;

d) the occurrence or non-occurrence of antidepressant-induced switch could be documented;

e) they were not rapid cyclers;

f) it was possible to demonstrate they had had definitely good or bad responses to the lithium prophylaxis.

The sample included 26 women and 25 men, with a mean age of onset of the disease of 32.9 ± 12.1 (SD) (range 12 to 59).

At time of starting lithium therapy, their ages were 17 to 65 (mean age 37.1 ± 13.3 SD), with a mean duration of illness of 67 ± 26 (SD) months.

Patients were considered to be switch-prone when at least one episode of drug-induced switching had occurred in the first four weeks of antidepressant treatment. Linking any mood swings to antidepressant treatment beyond this time would have been difficult, since all the patients had had prior episodes of mania and switches after a four-week treatment period could be natural relapses, not related to the therapy.

The criteria used to classify patients as lithium responders or non-responders were as follows: responders had no major affective relapses during the duration of treatment; non-responders had at least one affective episode meeting DSM 3 criteria for definite major affective disorder, not concomitant with a decrease in serum lithium levels to below 0.6 mmol/L and requiring supplementary medication with antidepressants or neuroleptics. Therefore, any patient who might somehow have benefited from lithium treatment, but for whom the benefit was not clearly discernible and who relapsed during treatment was not included in the analysis.We chose these rather conservative criteria of classification because we wished to characterize a subgroup of patients as precisely as possible.

RESULTS

Nineteen of 51 patients were switch-prone.

The sexes were distributed similarly in the two groups of switch-prone and non-switch-prone patients: 8 women and 11 men were switch-prone, 18 women and 14 men did not switch (chi square = 0.95; p = N.S.). The ratio of women who were menopausal to those who were non-menopausal at the onset of the disease and at the starting of lithium therapy was not significantly different in the two groups, though it was higher among switch-prone patients: 3/8 vs 1/17 (chi square 2.23; p = N.S.).

In the total population there were 24 lithium responders (47 %). Fifteen of the 19 switch-prone patients had poor outcome to the lithium prophylaxis, with only 4 having good responses, while in the group of patients who did not switch there were 20 lithium responders and 12 non-responders (chi square = 8.22; p <.005).

The specificity of the parameter switch-proneness for predicting a bad outcome to lithium prophylaxis is therefore 78.9 %, with the sensitivity 62.5 %, together yielding a correct classification of 68.6% (Table 1).

Table 1. Switch-proneness and lithium outcome.

SPECIFICITY	78.9%	FALSE POSITIVES	7.8%
SENSITIVITY	62.5%	FALSE NEGATIVES	23.5%
	CORRECT PREDICTION	68.6%	

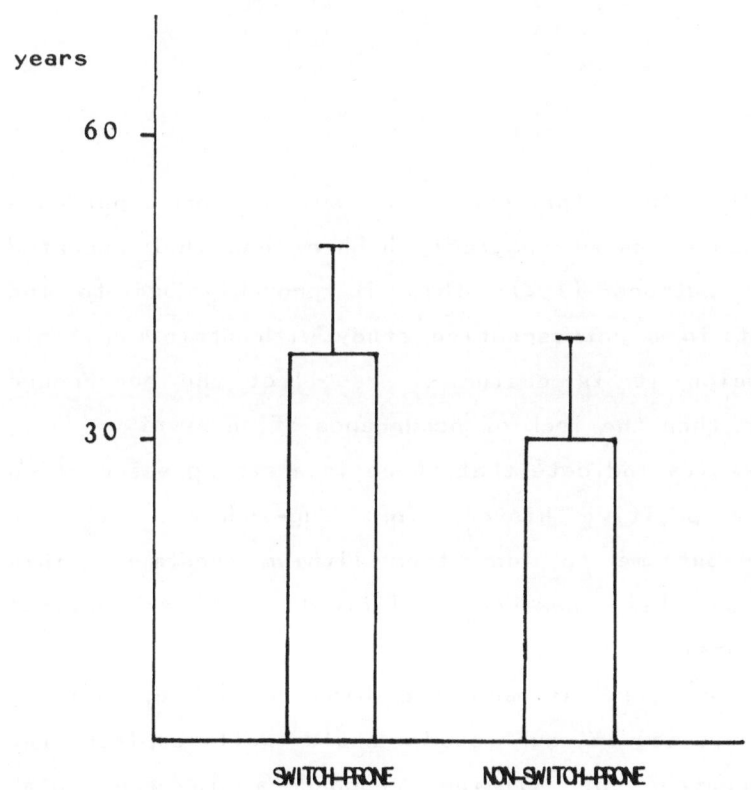

Figure 1. Age of onset of the disease for switch-prone and non-switch-prone patients.

While at the time when lithium therapy was started neither the age of the patients nor the duration of illness were different in the two groups, switch-prone patients had a higher age of onset of the disease than patients who did not switch: 38.3 ± 10.6 (SD) vs 29.7 ± 10.2 (SD); Student two tailed t test = 2.02; $p < .05$; (Fig. 1).

There were no differences between lithium responders and non-responders or between patients who did or did not switch in the mean number of affective episodes per year before lithium prophylaxis; the mean serum lithium levels were the same in responders and non-responders.

COMMENT

Undoubtedly the incidence of switch-prone patients in our study was unexpectedly higher than that reported by other authors (1,2); this is probably due to the fact that in a retrospective study with strict criteria of inclusion it is easier to recollect the occurrence of rather than the lack of occurrence of an event.

Our results indicate that there is a strong association between a positive history for drug-induced switching and poor outcome to long term lithium treatment. This association has numerous clinical and theoretical implications.

First of all, it and the high number of switch-prone patients in our study could well explain the low percentage of lithium responders in the total group of patients we studied. If the incidence of switch-proneness in our sample had been as low as that in other studies (1,2) the rate of lithium responders would have been similar to those generally reported in the literature (5).

From the clinical point of view, the occurrence of drug-induced switches seems to be a remarkably specific predictor for a negative response to long term lithium prophylaxis. It must be pointed out, however, that in our sample the sensitivity of this variable was not equal to its specificity in predicting the outcome of the lithium prophylaxis, with the sensitivity being lower than the specificity. Therefore, while the occurrence of a drug-induced switch is a useful tool for predicting a bad outcome to the lithium prophylaxis, the clinical usefulness of non-occurrence of the drug-induced switch does not necessarily imply a good outcome to the long term lithium treatment.This means that factors other than switch-proneness participate in determining a negative response to lithium prophylaxis and are responsible for the unequal powers of sensitivity and specificity of prediction.

However, it must be emphasized that the clinical usefulness of a variable is directly related to its incidence in the population. Therefore, further studies are required to get a better estimate of the incidence of switch-proneness in the Italian population before we can more precisely evaluate its usefulness in clinical practice as a predictor of lithium outcome.

From a more theoretical point of view, the difference in response to lithium prophylaxis is a first indication that the two groups of patients (those who do and those who do not switch) are different.

In line with our finding of a substantial ineffectiveness of lithium for prevention of affective recurrences in switch-prone patients, some previous studies (3,7) but not another (2), have reported that lithium is not efficacious in antagonizing drug-induced switches into mania; the inability of lithium to prevent both drug-induced switches and spontaneous recurrences in switch-prone patients suggests that a common pathogen-etic substrate underlies these mood swings and probably differentiates switch-prone patients from other lithium responding bipolar patients.

On the other hand, the hypothesis that some different mechanism underlies switch-proneness has been suggested (8) because the occurrence of the switch is independent of the duration of antidepressant treatment and of the type and dosage of antidepressant used (1).

Coming to a more detailed analysis of the variables that may be involved in producing our results, the pharmacological validation of switch-prone patients as a distinct subgroup of bipolar disorder does not seem to be influenced by the number of affective episodes nor by the age, the duration of illness at the start of lithium prophylaxis, or serum lithium levels: all these variables were, in fact, distributed randomly among the switch-prone and non-switch-prone patients.

Even the sex distribution in our two groups of patients were similar: this does not support the suggest-ion that sex hormones may be involved in the expression of drug-induced switch (3,7). Moreover, the higher ratio of menopausal women to non-menopausal women in the group of switch-prone patients further supports the concept that sex hormone cyclicity does not facilitate the development of drug-induced mania.

In addition, none of these variables seemed to be of importance to the lithium effectiveness in major affective disorder (9), independently of the occurrence or non-occurrence of switches.

On the contrary, the age of onset of the disease was different in switch-prone and non switch-prone patients. Switch-prone patients had a later age of onset than patients who did not switch. The mean age of onset of these latter patients (29.2) was quite similar to that generally reported for bipolar patients (10), whereas patients who switched had ages of onset whose mean (38.2) was shifted towards values more typical for unipolar patients. Interestingly, in a study of unipolar patients (11) it was shown that patients who had a drug-induced switch into mania had later ages of onset than patients who did not switch. This apparently greater vulnerability to drug-induced switch in patients with late onset major affective disorder could suggest the possibility that the mechanism(s) underlying the disease are somehow more easily destabilized in these patients than in early onset patients.

The finding that the age of onset was greater for the group of patients who were switch-prone and tended to not respond to lithium prophylaxis is consistent with some previous data of ours (9) that indicated that bipolar patients with late ages of onset have worse prognosis on lithium prophylaxis than patients with early ages of onset. However, the similarities of the percentages of poor responders among early ($<$ 40 yr) and late ($>$ 40 yr) onset patients support the idea that the association between switch-proneness and poor lithium prognosis is not merely a second order one, mediated by a later age of onset of switch-prone patients.

The difference in age of onset in the two groups of patients further strengthens the hypothesis that we are dealing with a distinct subgroup of patients:in fact, the variable "age of onset", like the variable "homogeneity of response to a particular therapy",has been claimed before to be a useful tool for clustering homogeneous subgroups of patients (4).

Therefore, two independent strategies provide support for the same hypothesis of the difference of switch-prone patients from bipolar patients who do not switch.

In conclusion, switch-proneness may be utilized as a nosological marker that is able to predict a bad outcome to the lithium prophylaxis and to identify a subgroup of patients with peculiar clinical and, possibly, biological characteristics, who could better benefit from some other prophylactic treatment. The definitive validation of the hypothesis that switch-proneness identifies a distinct subgroup of bipolar patients requires not only replication of our data with larger samples, but also biological and genetic studies specifically aimed at testing whether switch-prone patients have specific and homogeneous biological backgrounds and familial patterns.

REFERENCES

1. Bunney, W.E.Jr. (1978). Psychopharmacology of the switch process in affective illness. In: Lipton,M. Di Mascio,A., Killam,K.F.(eds). Psychopharmacology:A Generation of Progress. pp. 1249-1259. (New York:RavenPress)

2 . Lewis,J.L. and Winokur, G. (1982). The induction of mania. Arch.Gen.Psichiatry 39, 303-6
3. Quitkin,F.M., Kane,J., Rifkin,A., Ramos-Lorenzi,J.R., Nayak,D.V. (1981). Prophylactic lithium carbonate with and without imipramine for bipolar 1 patients. Arch.Gen.Psychiatry 38, 902-7
4.   Goodwin,F.K.,Cowdry,R.W.,Webster,M.H.   (1978). Predictors of drug-response in the affective disorders: towards an integrated approach. In: Lipton,M. et al (eds). Psychopharmacology:A generation of Progress. pp. 1277-1288. (New York: Raven Press)
5.   Gerbino,L.,   Oleshansky,M.,   Gershon,M.   (1978). Clinical use and mode of action of lithium. In: Lipton,M. et al. (eds). Psychopharmacology:A Generation of Progress. pp. 1261-1275. (New York: Raven Press)
6.   Cazzullo,   C.L.   and   Sacchetti,E.   Critical issues in the evaluation of long term lithium treatment.This book.
7. Wehr,T.A. and Goodwin,F.K. (1979). Rapid cycling in manic-depressive illness induced by tricyclic anti-depressants. Arch.Gen.Psychiatry 36, 555-9
8. Waters,G.H. and LaPierre,Y.D. (1982). Therapeutic use of the tricyclic-induced switch in bipolar manic-depression. Am.J.Psychiatry 139, 225-6
9. Sacchetti,E., Faravelli,C., Conte,G., Pennati,A., Vita,A., Cazzullo,C.L. (1983) Monoaminergic profiles in major affective disorders and clinical response to long term lithium treatment. Submitted for publication.
10 . Winokur,G. (1978). Mania and depression:family studies and genetics in relation to treatment. In:Lipton,M et al (eds). Psychopharmacology:A Generation of Progress. pp. 1213-1221. (New York:Raven Press)
11. van Scheyen,J.D. and van Kammen,D.P. (1979). Clomipramine-induced mania in unipolar depression. Arch.Gen.Psychiatry 36, 560-5

ACKNOWLEDGEMENTS

This research has been supported by the CNR contract N° 82.02298.56 to Dr. E.Sacchetti

Part IV
Clinical Aspects
of Long-term
Rubidium Treatment

17
Rubidium salts in depressed patients. An open pilot study using standardized techniques

P. SARTTESCHI, G. F. PLACIDI, A. LENZI, E. RAMPELLO AND G. B. CASSANO

The history of the therapeutic use in psychiatry of Rubidium strictly parallels that of Lithium. Both of these monovalent cations were employed during the 19th century in several pathological conditions, but not in mental illnesses, despite the very early observations of Lithium's sedative and hypnotic activity and of an elating effect of Rubidium in cardiopathic patients (1).

In the late sixties an interest in Rubidium reappeared after the effectiveness of Lithium in the treatment and prophylaxis of manic-depressive patients had been demonstrated. In 1969 Meltzer et al. (2) reported that Rubidium chloride had effects that were the opposite of those produced by Lithium; according to these authors, Rubidium increased the frequency of the EEG and behavioural activity in monkeys.

Soon afterwards, Stolk et al. (1970) (3) seemed to confirm, at a biochemical level, that Rubidium could be viewed as "anti-Lithium", since this cation seemed to increase the release of neuronally stored Norepinefrine (NE),

enhancing the 0-methylation pathway, while Lithium was
reported to increase the uptake of NE into synaptosomes
(4).

Such observations suggested that Rubidium could be
therapeutic for depression, as Lithium is for mania. More
recently a certain number of data have been made available
on its pharmacological and biochemical similarities with
classical antidepressant drugs, and its biological profile
is gradually becoming better defined.

Rubidium increases spontaneous motor activity and
antagonizes the effect of hypnotics in the same way as
Amphetamine (5). Like tricyclic-treated animals, Rubidium-
treated ones show an increased level of shock-elicited
aggressive behaviour and an increase in hyperactivity
induced by morphine, unlike Lithium, which decreases both.
Like most antidepressants, Rubidium increases noradrenergic
and dopaminergic transmission, but does not show any effect
on MAO and COMT activity, on adrenergic, serotoninergic,
GABAergic or colinergic receptors (6). Unlike Lithium, it
does not decrease Adenylcyclase activity (7).

Polygraphic EEG-sleep studies have shown that Rubidium
salts do not modify the REM stage, while they reduce stages
3 and 4 and increase 1 and 2, with a pattern similar to
that of tricyclics and amphetamine, which, however, reduce
the REM stage. As regards Lithium, controversial results
are reported in the literature; some authors have found a
decrease in REM and stage 4 (8), while others have observed
an increase in these stages (9).

Rubidium seems to act at a cellular level on membrane
transport in particular primarily affecting the
intracellular potassium metabolism, while Lithium produces
its major effect on the sodium metabolism. From biochemical

and pharmacological studies it appears that Rubidium may be essentially defined in negative terms as an "anti-Lithium" compound, even if it retains some characteristics similar to tricyclics and amphetamines; considering all these characteristics, it is hard to include Rubidium in any of the known categories of psychotropic drugs.

The clinical profile of Rubidium has still not been exactly defined, as its antidepressant or amphetamine-like effect is under discussion and uncertain. The possible clinical activity of Rubidium has been investigated in only a very few studies. Interest on this topic was stimulated by the first observations of Meltzer and Fieve (2,10,11,12,13) who observed an improvement in a high percentage of patients.

These studies have also elucidated the pharmacokinetic profile of Rubidium, which is rapidly and completely absorbed after oral administration, reaching its maximum plasma level within 60-90 minutes. Its intracellular penetration is very slow and the ratio between intra-erythrocyte and plasma Rubidium, in physiological conditions, is about 20-30. Higher values may be quite critical, since they may represent possible toxic levels. The metal becomes distributed in the liver and muscles but only very slowly in the central nervous system: it is eliminated very slowly mainly by the kidney and its half-life ranges from 30 to 60 days.

Other studies (14, 15, 16) reported an improvement in depressive patients belonging to different categories.

In a single blind study in which Rubidium was compared with imipramine, it was reported that the salt improved 65% of depressive patients, acting in particular on psychomotor retardation (17). No toxic or side effects were observed and no correlation was found between clinical improvement and plasma levels of Rubidium.

Moreover, a slight improvement in akynisia in Parkinsonian patients (18) and in motor retardation and emotional withdrawal in schizophrenics (19) has been observed after Rubidium treatment; however, an increase in hostility and persecutory delusions were observed in psychotic subjects treated with higher doses of the salt.

It has been also noticed (20) that the cycles of manic depressive patients treated with Rubidium Chloride decrease in duration and severity, with prolonged manic episodes and shorter depressive episodes.

In the only double-blind study (21), up to day reported Rubidium appeared superior to Chlorimipramine. No particular side effects were reported and the therapeutic effect was related to plasma levels of Rubidium ranging from 0.102 to 0.320 mEq/l. Although promising results have been reported by various authors, comparison between them is difficult because of the different methodologies adopted.

The aim of this investigation was to evaluate the effect of Rubidium in depressive disorders in an open pilot study using standardized techniques.

We consider such a study to be the necessary condition to future investigation of a compound that has been as little investigated as Rubidium.

MATERIAL AND METHOD

Patients

Twenty-one newly admitted depressed female inpatients aged 21-75 years were admitted to the study. The diagnosis was made according to DSM-III.

Patients showing conditions such as organic brain

damage, cardiovascular disease, alcoholism, drug abuse, and pregnancy were excluded.

Experimental design

A wash-out period (2-3 days)was followed by an open trial lasting 3 weeks. During this the patients were given Rubidium Chloride in a flexible dosage schedule ranging from a minimum of 180 mg to a maximum of 540 mg. Each capsule contained 180 mg. Since Rubidium seems to possess activating and disinhibiting properties without sleep-inducing effects, a benzodiazepine - Lorazepam (7.5-15 mg.) - was the only concomitant drug allowed.

Assessment instruments

Prior to treatment demographic data were collected using the Adult Personal Data Inventory (APDI). Before treatment started, and at weekly intervals thereafter the symptomatology was evaluated with the following rating devices: Clinical Global Improvement (CGI), Hamilton Depression Scale (HAM-D), Hamilton Anxiety Scale (HAM-A), Brief Psychiatric Rating Scale (BPRS) and Self-Administered Depression Scale (SADS). Dosage and side-effects were recorded using Dosage and Treatment Emergent Symptoms Scale (DOTES) and Tess Write In Scale (TWIS) weekly and at any dosage change.

This battery (with exception of the APDI) and the Patient Termination Record (PTR) was used whenever the patient stopped treatment.

The data were analyzed at the CCPDD of the Institute of Clinical Psychiatry of Pisa University by means of the standard procedures of BLIPS/BDP and the non-standard routines of BMDP.

Laboratory examinations

Prior to commencement and at the end of the treatment, the following examinations were carried out: complete blood count, serum glutamic oxalacetic transaminase (SGOT), serum glutamic piruvic transaminase (SGPT), blood urea nitrogen, serum glucose, gamma-GT, alkaline phosphatase, creatinine, bilirubine, electrolytes.

The blood levels of Rubidium were determined by Atomic Absorption Spectrophotometry according to Sutter et al. (22).

In six patients who terminated the trial, EKG was performed before starting and at the end of the treatment.

RESULTS

Personal data (APDI)

21 female inpatients were admitted to the trial. Their mean age was 56.95 years. Adopting DSM-III criteria, the most common diagnosis on the first axis was Major depression (recurrent) (43.3%), followed by Dysthymic (28.2%), Cyclothymic (14%) and Bipolar disorders (14.5%) (depressive) (Tab. 1).

Termination data (PTR)

The mean duration of the treatment was 15 days (Tab. 2). Nine (47.6%) of 21 patients terminated the 21 day trial.

Premature terminations were due to adverse reactions (9.5%) (1 case of   diarrhea, 1 case of increase of SGPT and SGOT) and ineffectiveness in 5 patients (23%).

As their condition had improved, some patients asked to be discharged, and six of them did not return for the following weekly evaluation.

Dosage data

The minimum and maximum daily doses given were 180 mg

TABLE 1-PATIENTS' DIAGNOSTIC FEATURES (DSM-III)

I AXIS (CLINICAL SYNDROMES)		
MAJOR DEPRESSION (RECURRENT)	10	(47.7%)
DYSTHYMIC DISORDER (DEPRESSIVE NEUROSIS)	6	(28.6%)
CYCLOTHYMIC DISORDER	3	(14.2%)
BIPOLAR DISORDER (DEPRESSIVE)	2	(9.5%)

II AXIS (PERSONALITY DISORDERS)			
HISTRIONIC	8	(38.1%)	AVOIDANT 1 (4.8%)
PARANOID	2	(9.5%)	COMPULSIVE 1 (4.8%)
DEPENDENT	2	(9.5%)	NONE 7 (33.3%)

III AXIS (ORGANIC DISEASES)			
ABSENT	18	(85.6%)	CHRONIC HEPATITIS 1 (4.8%)
HYPOTHYROIDISM	1	(4.8%)	TRIGEMINAL PAIN 1 (4.8%)

IV AXIS (PRECIPITATING EXTERNAL STRESSOR)			
ABSENT	11	(52.4%)	
PROBABLY PRESENT	7	(33.3%)	DEFINITELY PRESENT 3 (14.2%)

V AXIS (SOCIAL FUNCTIONING DURING THE LAST YEAR)			
ADEQUATE	11	(52.4%)	MARKED DECLINE 1 (4.8%)
SOME DECLINE	6	(28.6%)	FLUCTUATING 3 (14.2%)

TABLE 2- PATIENT   TERMINATION RECORD

TOTAL NO. OF PATIENTS	21
TOTAL DAYS IN STUDY:	
MEAN	15.00 (± 5.97)
PREMATURE TERMINATION	
ADVERSE REACTION	2 (9.5%)
INEFFECTIVENESS	4 (19.0%)
PATIENT DID NOT RETURN	6 (28.5%)
TOTAL PREMATURE TERMINATIONS	12 (57.2%)
NOT PREMATURELY TERMINATED	9 (42.8%)
DRUG INTAKE	
NO IRREGULARITIES	21
ANY IRREGULARITIES	0

Lorazepam was given at daily dosages ranging from 7.5 to 15 mg. and administered daily and nightly throughout the duration of the trial.

Efficacy data

CGI. During treatment with Rubidium, the score for Severity of Illness" decreased significantly from a mean initial value of 4.48 (intermediate between "moderate" and "marked") to a final one of 3.86 (close to "moderate").

The global improvement score at the end of trial was 2.89 (close to "minimally improved") (Tab. 3). 13 patients (61.9%) showed improvement. It is interesting to note that improvement was greatest during the second week (15 patients); thereafter 2 of the improved patients worsened. HAM-D. The data obtained with the HAM-D have been analyzed according to the factorialization suggested by Cleary and Guy (23) (Tab. 4). The factors "retardation" and "loss of

TABLE 3—EVALUATION OF GENERAL IMPROVEMENT IN PATIENTS WITH RUBIDIUM SALTS

		MEAN SCORE
CGI		
SEVERITY OF ILLNESS	INITIAL	4.48 (BETWEEN "MODERATE" AND "MARKED") (*)
	FINAL	3.86 (CLOSE TO "MODERATE")
GLOBAL IMPROVEMENT		2.89 (CLOSE TO "MINIMALLY IMPROVED")
NO. OF PATIENTS IMPROVED		13 (61.90%)

(*) F VALUE 5.97
    p <.01

TABLE 4—HAM-D FACTORS (*) : NO. AND % OF SYMPTOMATIC PATIENTS IMPROVED AND RESULTS OF VARIANCE ANALYSIS

FACTORS	NO. OF SYMPTOMATIC PATIENTS	SYMPTOMATIC PATIENTS IMPROVED		ANALYSIS OF VARIANCE			
		NO.	%	INITIAL	FINAL	F VALUE	p
ANXIETY SOMATIZATION	21	4	19.05	1.28	1.04	2.90	-
WEIGHT LOSS	14	9	64.29	1.37	0.62	9.00	<.01
COGNITIVE DISTURBANCE	21	3	14.29	1.01	0.75	4.31	-
DIURNAL VARIATION	17	8	42.06	1.80	1.10	3.20	-
SLEEP DISTURBANCE	20	7	35.00	1.94	2.59	1.62	-
RETARDATION	21	8	38.1	2.42	1.91	5.49	<.01
TOTAL SCORE				23.05	17.62	9.23	<.01

(*) CLEARY AND GUY (1975)

weight" were significantly reduced at the end of the trial. The total score of the same rating instrument also decreased significantly.

HAM-A. The analysis of the two factors "Somatic" and "Psychic Anxiety" (24) demonstrated a significant fall in the scores of both factors, and in the total score (Tab. 5).

SADS. Variance analysis on the SADS items demonstrate a statistically significant fall in the scores of almost all the items expressing depressive symptomatology, and of some items which are most closely related to anxiety (Tab. 6).

BPRS. The BPRS scale was analyzed both on single items and on the factor scores (25) (Tab. 7). All the items exploring depressive and anxious symptomatology were rated as present at the beginning of the treatment; whereas the item "Suspiciousness" was present in only 8 of the 21 patients. The items which seem to respond to this treatment were "Depressive Mood" (13 patients, 61.4%), "Motor Retardation" (12 patients, 63.2%) and "Blunted Affect" (11 patients, 52.4%) and the factor which showed the greatest improvement seemed to be "Anxiety-Depression" (10 patients, 47.6%).

In addition, the items "Suspiciousness" and "Tension" and the factor "Hostil·-Suspiciousness" appear to be significantly influenced by the treatment.

Side effect data

Analysis of side effects rated with the DOTES and TWIS scales did not indicate the presence of severe side effects; as regards the moderate ones, one case of diarrhea, one of slight confusional state, and two cases of pollakiuria were observed. Mild symptoms were present in many patients (Tab. 8), but were not disturbing enough to

TABLE 5—HAM-A FACTORS (*): NO. AND % OF SYMPTOMATIC PATIENTS IMPROVED
AND RESULTS OF VARIANCE ANALYSIS

FACTORS	NO. OF SYMPTOMATIC PATIENTS	PATIENTS IMPROVED		ANALYSIS OF VARIANCE			
		NO.	%	INITIAL SCORE	FINAL SCORE	F VALUE	p
SOMATIC ANXIETY	21	4	19.05	1.09	0.80	6.55	<.01
PSYCHIC ANXIETY	21	8	38.10	1.71	1.28	12.81	<.01
TOTAL SCORE	21	7	35.33	19.62	14.57	12.20	<.01

(*) HAMILTON (1959)

TABLE 6

SADS (SELF-ADMINISTERING DEPRESSION SCALE): RESULT OF VARIANCE ANALYSIS. ONLY ITEMS SIGNIFICANTLY DECREASED DURING RUBIDIUM TREATMENT ARE REPORTED.

	MEAN SCORE		F VALUE	p
	INITIAL	FINAL		
1. DEPRESSIVE MOOD	3.33	2.67	6.48	<.01
3. CRYING	2.52	1.76	2.49	<.05
7. LOSS OF WEIGHT	1.87	1.62	5.65	<.01
8. CONSTIPATION	2.90	2.28	5.68	<.01
9. TACHYCARDIA	2.14	1.57	2.06	<.01
10. ASTHENIA	3.52	2.52	2.42	<.01
11. INABILITY CONCENT.	2.95	2.33	1.66	<.05
12. INABILITY WORK	3.33	2.95	2.07	<.05
13. ANXIETY PSYCHIC	3.09	2.33	2.53	<.01
14. HOPELESSNESS	3.00	2.38	3.61	<.05
17. NO MEAN IN LIFE	3.38	2.48	3.15	<.01
26. INNER SHAKINESS	2.90	2.28	3.48	<.01
29. REMAINING IN BED	3.14	2.00	2.02	<.05
31. SUBJECTIVE RATING OF SEVERITY	3.29	2.80	4.04	<.01
TOTAL SCORE	80.81	65.85	9.22	<.01

TABLE 7-NO. AND % OF PATIENTS IMPROVED IN BPRS ITEMS AND FACTORS. RESULTS OF VARIANCE ANALYSIS. ONLY ITEMS AND FACTORS RELATED TO THE DEPRESSION ARE REPORTED.

	NO. OF PATIENTS RATED SYMPTO. AT PRE-DRUG	NO. OF PATIENTS RATED IMPROVED		MEAN SCORE		F VALUE	p
	NO.	NO.	PER CENT	INITIAL	FINAL		
BPRS ITEMS							
SOMATIC CONCERN	18	9	50.0	3.00	2.52	2.10	-
ANXIETY	21	7	53.3	3.81	3.48	2.05	-
GUILT FEELINGS	12	7	58.3	2.10	1.76	1.52	-
TENSION	12	9	75.0	1.95	1.43	4.57	<.01
DEPRESSIVE MOOD	21	13	61.9	4.76	3.67	13.32	<.01
SUSPICIOUSNESS	8	8	100.0	1.71	1.05	10.00	<.01
MOTOR RETARDAT.	19	12	63.2	2.81	2.00	9.41	<.01
BLUNTED AFFECT	19	11	52.4	2.38	1.90	5.52	<.01
BPRS FACTORS							
ANXIETY DEPRESSION	21	10	47.6	3.42	2.86	7.91	<.01
ANERGIA	18	7	34.8	1.77	1.50	6.78	<.01
HOSTIL. SUSPICIOUSNESS	9	7	77.7	1.24	1.02	9.97	<.01

TABLE 8- SIDE EFFECT DATA (DOTES AND TWIS)	MILD	MOD.	SEV.	TOT.
ANTI-CHOLINERGIC				
DROWSINESS	5	0	0	5
DRY MOUTH	1	0	0	1
BLURRED VISION	4	0	0	4
TOTAL SYMPTOMS				10 (18%)
CENTRAL NERVOUS SYSTEM				
RIGIDITY	2	0	0	2
TREMOR	1	0	0	1
DYSTONIC SYMPTOMS	1	0	0	1
AKATHISIA	1	0	0	1
TOTAL SYMPTOMS				5 (9%)
NEUROTIC				
INSOMNIA	2	0	0	2
CONSTIPATION	1	0	0	1
WEIGHT LOSS	3	0	0	3
HEADACHE	5	0	0	5
TOTAL SYMPTOMS				11 (20%)
AUTONOMIC NERVOUS SYSTEM				
DIARRHEA	5	1	0	6
TOTAL SYMPTOMS				6 (11%)
DELIRIUM				
TOXIC CONFUSIONAL STATE	4	1	0	5
EXCITEMENT/AGITATION	3	0	0	3
TOTAL SYMPTOMS				8 (14%)
ABNORMAL LABORATORY FINDINGS				
ABNORMAL LIVER	1	0	0	1
ABNORMAL URINE	0	2	0	2
TOTAL SYMPTOMS				3 (5%)
MISCELLANEOUS (INCLUDING TWIS)				
INCREASED MOTOR ACTIVITY	1	0	0	1
DECREASED MOTOR ACTIVITY	1	0	0	1
SWEATING	3	0	0	3
HYPERTENSION	1	0	0	1
WEIGHT GAIN	5	0	0	5
ANOREXIA/DECR. APPETITE	2	0	0	2
TOTAL SYMPTOMS				13 (23%)
TOTAL SYMPTOMS			56	

justify stopping the treatment.

Laboratory data

In the six patients, whose EKG was recorded at the beginning and at end of trial, the only parameter showing a significant change was heart rate, which showed a fall all the cases studied (Tab. 9). As regards the changes specific to hyperkalemia, they were present in about 30% of our cases, but they were so slight as not to be indicative of real hyperkalemia.

Laboratory data showed no significant differences between initial and final values.

Rubidium blood levels were between 1.5-3.7 mEq/l and no correlations were found between blood concentrations and clinical improvement.

DISCUSSION

The purpose of the present trial was to evaluate in an open pilot study the clinical effects of Rubidium Salts by utilizing a combination of widely accepted international rating scales processed by advanced computer techniques. This made it possible to obtain a systematic and comprehensive documentation of the trial and to facilitate general comprehension of the data, so yielding important gains in the methodology of clinical trial execution.

The results of this open trial indicated that Rubidium Chloride was effective in a quite large percentage (61.9%) of our patients.

Premature termination due to rapid improvement included six patients who did not return to complete the trial. There were six (28.6%) non-responders (stationary or worsened) and in 2 patients (9.5%) the treatment was interrupted because of adverse reactions.

TABLE 9

EFFECTS OF RUBIDIUM SALTS ON SOME EKG PARAMETERS EVALUATED BEFORE (I) AND AFTER (II) THE TREATMENT

CODE NO.	HEART RATE/MIN		PR INTERVAL (SEC)		QRS DURATION (SEC)		QI INTERVAL (SEC)	
	I	II	I	II	I	II	I	II
503	85	73	0.15	0.15	0.09	0.08	0.35	0.34
504	94	89	0.19	0.17	0.08	0.08	0.36	0.38
505	91	84	0.16	0.17	0.07	0.08	0.35	0.35
507	84	61	0.18	0.19	0.08	0.09	0.32	0.39
508	98	89	0.14	0.14	0.08	0.08	0.32	0.34
518	69	53	0.16	0.17	0.07	0.08	0.41	0.45

CHANGES IN SOME EKG INDEXES OF HYPERPOTASSEMIA DURING RUBIDIUM TREATMENT

CODE NO.	HIGHEST AND SHARPEST T WAVE	R WAVE DIMINISHMENT	QRS ENLARGEMENT	PROGRESSIVE DECREASE IN P WAVE HEIGHT
503	-	-	-	-
504	-	-	-	-
505	+	+	+	+
507	-	-	-	-
508	-	-	-	-
518	+	+	-	-

The mean period that elapsed before significant improvement was observed   between 7 and 15 days .

Besides revealing the significant fall in the total score of all rating devices employed in this study, variance analysis made it possible to isolate some factors and items which showed a marked fall.

In particular, the greatest significant effects exerted by Rubidium seem to be those exerted on the "Retardation" and "Loss of Weight" factors in the HAM-D scale, and on the "Anxiety/Depression", "Anergia", and "Hostility-Suspiciousness" factors and the "Depressive Mood", "Motor Retardation", "Blunted Affect", "Tension" and "Suspiciousness" items in the BPRS scale. This trend towards improvement seems to be confirmed by SADS, which showed a statistically significant fall in almost all the items exploring depressive symptomatology and in some of the items most closely related to anxiety.

As regards analysis of the factors and items most typical of anxiety, it has to be pointed out that in all our patients Lorazepam was used as concomitant medication, since Rubidium was known to have stimulating properties (2) without sedating and sleep-inducing effects. For this reason it was not possible in this study to evaluate the effect of this compound on anxiety symptoms.

The side effects registered with DOTES and TWIS were not severe Treatment need to be stopped in two patients, in one case because of diarrhe a which was rated as moderate, and in the other because of an increase in SGOT and SGPT in a patient with previous chronic hepatit is.

During Rubidium treatment, the six EKG monitored patients showed only a lowering of heart rate with no clear-cut EKG signs of hyperkaliema.

In conclusion, even if it is not possible to obtain definite data from this open pilot study, our results seem to confirm previous clinical observations of an activity of this substance on depressive illness. The effect of Rubidium on "Retardation", which has been considered "the specific emotional response which defines the core of depression" (26) is of special interest. From BPRS analysis profiles it is possible to hypothesize that this compound may be most effective in a subgroup of depressive disorders grouped by Overall (27) under the heading "hostile depression". In our sample, in fact, besides the most typical items in depression such as "Depressive Mood", "Motor Retardation", and "Blunted Affect", which all showed a significant fall in total score, the item "Suspiciousness" appears to be strongly influenced by treatment, so much so that all the patients rated as symptomatic at beginning of treatment showed improvement.

Our data on the frequency and severity of unwanted effects and laboratory findings indicate a high degree of tolerability for Rubidium Salts.

On the basis of the clinical information now available, including that gathered in the present trial, it appears useful to plan further controlled studies against placebo and thereafter against active antidepressants. Such studies could aim to achieve a more accurate definition of its spectrum of activity, which - considering its pharmacologic characteristics - could be quite different from those of the most common antidepressant drugs.

REFERENCES

1. Botkin, S.S. (1888). The influence of the salts of Rubidium and Coesium upon the heart and circulation in connection with the laws physiological action of alkali metals. St. Petersburg Military Academy, Doctoral Dissertation.

2. Meltzer, H.L., Taylor, R.M., Platman, S.R., and Fieve, R.R. (1969). Rubidium: A potential modifier of affect and behavior. Nature,233, 321-322.

3. Stolk, J.M., Nowack, W.J., and Bargaas, J.D. (1970). Brain norepinephrine: enhanced turnover after rubidium treatment. Science, 168, 501-503.

4. Colburn, R., Goodwin, F., and Bonney, W.E. Jr (1967). Effect of Lithium on the uptake of noradrenaline by synaptosomes. Nature, 215, 1395-1397.

5. Simon, P. (1978). Que peut apporter la pharmacologie experimentale à l'étude des antidépresseurs? In: Pichot, P. (eds). Les voyes nouvelles de la dépression pp. 162-168 (Paris: Masson).

6. Gessa, G.L. (1983). Unpublished results.

7. Wang, Y.C., Pandey, G.N., Mendels, J., and Frazer, A. (1974). Effect of Lithium on prostaglandin E1 stimulated adenylate cyclase of human platelets. Biochem. Pharmacol., 4, 845.

8. Kupfer, D.J., Wyatt, R.G., Greenspan, K., and Snyder, F. (1970). Lithium carbonate and sleep in affective illness. Arch. Gen. Psychiat., 23, 261-268.

9. Maggini, C., Andreoli, V., and Guazzelli, M. (1975). Studio poligrafico del sonno in maniaci ed ipomaniaci trattati con carbonato di Litio. Riv. Neurol., 45, 209-216.

10. Meltzer, H.L., and Lubermann, K.W. (1971). Chronic ingestion of Rubidium without toxicity: implication for human therapy. Experientia, 6, 672.

11. Meltzer, H.L., and Fieve, R.R. (1975). Rubidium in psychiatry and medicine:an overview. In: Essman, W.B., and Valzelli, L. (eds). Current Developments in Psychopharmacology pp. 205-242. (Spectrum Publications, Inc.).

12. Fieve, R.R., Meltzer, H.L., and Taylor, R.M. (1971). Rubidium Chloride ingestion by volunteer subjects: initial experience. Psychopharmacologia, 4, 307-316.

13. Fieve, R.R., Meltzer, H.L., and Taylor, R.M. (1971). Mendlewicz, J., and Thomas, A. (1973). Rubidium: biochemical, behavioral and metabolic studies in humans. Am. J. Psychiat., 1 , 55-61.

14.Platman, S.R.(1971). Lithium and Rubidium. A role in the affective disorders. Dis. Nerv., 9, 604.

15. Torregiani, G. (1972). Unpublished results (personal comunication).

16. Sacco, F. (1972). Unpublished results (personal communication).

17. Carolei, A., Sonsini, V., Casacchia, M., Agnoli, A., and Fazio, C. (1975). Azione farmacologica del cloruro di Rubidio. Effetto antidepressivo: confronto con l'Imipramina. Clin. Terap., 75, 469-478.

18. Casacchia, M., Carolei, A., Zamponi, A., Meco, G., and Agnoli, A. (1975). Cloruro di Rubidio e morbo di Parkinson, dati preliminari. Acta Neurol., 30, 615-618.

19. Chouinard, G. and, Annable, L. (1977). The effect of Rubidium in schizophrenia. Comm. Psychopharmacol., 1,

373-383.

20. Paschalis, C., Jenner, F.A., and LEE, C.R. (1978). Effects of rubidium chloride on the course of manic-depressive illness. J. Ray. Soc. Med., 71, 343-352.

21. Calandra, C., and Nicolosi, M. (1980). Confronto fra due farmaci ad azione antidepressiva: Rubidio cloruro e clorimipramina.Proceedings of 34th Congress of Italian Society of Psychiatry, Catania, Italy.

22. Sutter E., Platman S.R. and Fieve R.R. (1970). Atomic Absorption and Spectrophotometry of Rubidium in Biological Fluids. Clinical Chemistry, 16, 602-605.

23. Cleary, P., and Guy, W. (1977). Factor analyses of the Hamilton Depression Scale. Drugs Exptl. Clin. Res., 1, 115-120.

24. Hamilton, M. (1959). The assessment of anxiety status by rating. Brit. J. Med. Psychol., 32, 50-55.

25. Guy, W., Cleary, P., and Bonato, R.R. (1975). Methodological implication of a large central data symptom. Proceedings of IXth Congress CINP (Amsterdam) Excerpta Medica.

26. Vidlocher, D. (1983). Retardation: a basic emotional response? In: Davis, J.M., and Maas, J.W. (eds). The Affective Disorders. pp 165-181 (Washington: American Psychiatric Press, Inc.).

27. Overall, J. (1983). Phenomenological heterogeneity of depressive disorders. In: Davis, J.M., and Maas, J.W. (eds). The Affective Disorders. pp. 151-163. (Washington: American Psychiatric Press, Inc.).

18
Preliminary results with rubidium in depressed patients

G. U. CORSINI, M. REDA, C. BURRRAI, A. PODDIGHE AND N. RUDAS

Lithium and Rubidium are closely linked in their history as far as their the rapeutic use in psychiatry is concerned. The introduction of rubidium into human therapy during the 19th century was mainly directed towards the treatment of several pathological conditions, also including epilepsy and syphilis, but not mental illnesses, despite the early observation of Botkin (1). This author occasionally reported that several of his cardiac patients, treated with approximately 1.6g of rubidium showed a subjective feeling of well-being. Following this observation, 80 years passed before a controlled study on the psychiatric effects of rubidium was carried out. This study was undertaken as a consequence of the excellent results obtained with lithium in the therapy and prophylaxis of manic-depressive psychosis. It was shown that rubidium increased EEG frequency and behavioural activity in monkeys (2) and consequent to opposite results obtained with lithium, the authors suggested that rubidium might have a clinical application in the treatment of affective disorders. Subsequently, several observations led to the assumption that rubidium and lithium have opposite behavioural, electroencephalographic and biochemical properties (3,4,5,6,7,8), thus further defining the potential antidepressant activity of the former. The possible clinical activity of rubidium has been investigated by early studies of Meltzer and Fieve (9,10,11,12). These authors studied 25 depressed patients resistant to other treatments, affected by either unipolar or bipolar syndromes. The experimental design consisted of a cross-over study with placebo or rubidium for a period of 2 to 4 weeks. Blood rubidium levels reached 0.44 mEq/l. Positive response varied depending on the duration of treatment: 70% after 4 weeks, 57% after 3 weeks, 45% after 2 weeks. Subsequently, a single blind study in which rubidium was compared to imipramine was carried out (13). Thirty depressed patients (endogenous, reactive, neurotic or involutional) received rubidium chloride for 4 weeks at a maximum dosage of 540mg per day. The salt improved 65% of these patients, acting in particular on depressive mood and psychomotor retardation as well, and did not produce any specific side effects. Two studies on the effect of rubidium in chronic schizophrenics were carried out in Canada, at the McGill University (14,15). The treatment consisted of single administration of 1g of rubidium chloride in addition to the usual neuroleptic regimen. The results of these studies underlined a slight beneficial effect of the salt on emotional withdrawal and motor retardation without producing any toxic reaction or altering EEG, EKG, or routine laboratory tests.

Paschalis et al (16) reported in 5 rapid cyclic patients, resistant to other therapy, that rubidium decreases the duration and severity of dystimic phases but prolongs manic episodes.

247

More recently, in a double blind study, the only one so far reported, 28 depressed patients received rubidium chloride at the dosage of 540mg/day or chlorimipramine at 100mg/day for a period of 30 days. Rubidium appeared to be superior to chlorimipramine and no major side effects were noted (17). These clinical data, although with some limitations as to number and type of trial, suggest that rubidium might exert an antidepressant action with no relevant side effects and in order to further evaluate this suggestion we investigated the effects of this cation on depressed patients in an open pilot study and we report here the preliminary findings.

MATERIALS AND METHODS

Patients

Ten newly admitted depressed patients (6 males and 4 females) aged from 37 - 56 years were included in this study. All patients were selected on the basis of the Diagnostic Criteria for Affective Disorders as reported in the DSM III. Patients affected by pathological conditions such as organic brain syndromes, cardiovascular, hepatic and renal diseases and alcoholism, as well as pregnant subjects, were excluded.

The patients were assigned to an experimental group receiving rubidium chloride. Informed consent was obtained from all patients.

Experimental Design.

After a short wash-out period (2-4 days), all patients underwent an open trial lasting no longer than 4 weeks. After the inclusion in the experimental group, the patients received rubidium chloride (180mg per capsule) ranging from 1 to 3 capsules per day (minimum 180mg and maximum 540mg). A benzodiazepine, Lorazepam, from 1 to 2.5mg per day, was the only concomitant drug allowed.

Psychometric Assessments.

The Hamilton Depression Scale (HDS) was used throughout the study and was applied on admission (T_o), at day 7 (T_1), at day 14 (T_2), at day 21 (T_3) and at day 28 (T_4) of treatment. The patients were evaluated using the Beck self-rating Depression Scale (BSRDS) on admission and at the end of the trial. Side effects were recorded using the Treatment Emergent Symptoms Scale (TESS) once weekly. The score obtained was analyzed using Wilcoxon's signed rank test.

Laboratory Tests.

On admission and at the end of the trial, the following examinations were carried out: blood pressure, serum glucose, blood urea nitrogen, complete blood counts, serum glutamic piruvic transaminase (SGPT), serum glutamic oxalacetic transaminase, alkaline phosphatase, γ-GT, creatinine, bilirubine and electrolytes. EKG was carried out in all patients before and after the treatment.

RESULTS

Ten patients, as reported in Table 1, completed the study. Two additional patients, of whom the results are not reported, were admitted to the study but they did not complete it due to reasons unrelated to the drug treatment. One, a 33 year old female, refused to continue treatment after one week because she belived any therapeutic approach to be useless. The second, a 54 year old female, dropped out of the study after a few days of treatment since a more careful examination of her EKG, performed before the trial, revealed signs of miocardial ischemia. Both patients however, during drug administration, did not show any toxic effects related to the drug treatment.

Table 1 shows that major depression (recurrent) and dysthimic disorders were represented by 3 patients respectively and 2 out of ten were classified as having bipolar disorders of depressed type.

TABLE 1.

	Rubidium Chloride
Number of patients	10
male	6
female	4
mean age	47.4
range age	37 – 56
Diagnosis	
Bipolar disorder, depressed	2
Major depression, single episode	1
Major depression, recurrent	3
Cyclothymic disorder (depressive period)	1
Dysthymic disorder	3
Duration of treatment (weeks)	4
Daily dosage	180 – 540mg

HRS scores, reported in Table 2, show that after one week of treatment (T_1) there was a slight mean improvement (19.9%) of depressive symptoms. Only after 2 weeks (T_2) however did this improvement reach a statistically significant difference in respect to the initial value (T_o). After 3 and 4 weeks of

TABLE 2.

HRS SCORES

		RUBIDIUM CHLORIDE		
	Average	S.E.	%	P
T_o	28.2	1.1	–	–
T_1	22.6	1.5	–19.9	n.s
T_2	18.5	1.6	–34.4	<.01
T_3	15.3	1.9	–45.8	<.01
T_4	13.1	1.9	–53.6	<.01

% and P in respect to initial values.

treatment, the scores decreased further but to a lesser extent (45% – T_2 and 53.6% – T_4 respectively). Similarly, the BSRDS scores before (T_o) and after the study (T_4) showed a statistically significant difference with a decrease of 51.6% at T_4 (Table 3).

TABLE 3.

BSRDS SCORES

	Average	S.E.	%	P
T_o	34.5	3.5	–	–
T_4	16.7	2.6	–51.6	<.01

% and P in respect to initial values.

At the end of the trial, six patients were evaluated as having a "good" therapeutic outcome (bipolar disorder 1, major depression 3, dysthymic disorder 2). All of them were dismissed without specific therapy except for a benzo-diazepine (Lorazepam) and were periodically controlled. Four patients out of the six showed a good mental condition on further psychiatric control after one month. One patient out of the six did not return to further controls and the last one relapsed after about 3 weeks. The patients who presented "fair" (cyclothymic disorder 1, dysthymic disorder 1), "poor" (major depression 1) or "no change" (bipolar disorder, depressed) at the end of the study, were switched to a conventional antidepressant therapy. (Table 4).

TABLE 4.

Therapeutic outcome of patients under Rubidium Chloride	
	N° of patients
Good (> 50%)	6
Fair (< 50%)	2
Poor (< 25%)	1
No Change	1

HRS score evaluation at the end of the trial (T_4).

The improvement of the depressive symptomatology concerned all HRS items. The side effects occurring in the patients are shown in Table 5. One patient suffered episodes of headache, others were affected by: dry mouth (1), nausea (1), constipation (1), diarrhea (2) and gastric distress (1). All these effects were very slight and did not require interruption of the treatment. Blood pressure, heart rate and laboratory tests were all within the normal range at the end of the study.

TABLE 5.

Side effects during the treatment.	
	N° of patients
Headache	1
Dry Mouth	2
Nausea	1
Constipation	1
Diarrhea	2
Gastric distress	1

Itels already positive on admission were excluded.

DISCUSSION

In agreement with the data already reported in literature, the preliminary results of this open study suggest that Rubidium Chloride exerts an antidepressant action. However, the experimental design used and the scarce number of patients studied suggest that the results obtained should be considered with caution; infact, the open design was chosen as it was considered a necessary preliminary study for a more complex and in depth investigation. The number of patients allows a rather limited statistical study, even though it indicates therapeutical efficacy and low toxicity. Moreover, the length of treatment (4 weeks) was chosen on the basis of previous experience present in the literature and was not prolonged further due to kinetical considerations of the compound. Infact, Rubidium possesses a rather long biological half-life and therefore this cation tends to accumulate in the organism, rendering problematical prolonged treatment. The daily dose of Rubidium Chloride (180-540mg) used in this study was decided on according to data concerning the efficacy and non-toxicity present in literature.

Even with these limitations, it is possible to form several considerations concerning the results obtained: the improvement of depressive symptomatology in our patients was gradual but showed therapeutical efficacy after only 2 weeks of treatment. Further treatment led to a mean improvement of more than 50% which was considered as being fairly good. This improvement concerned all items of the Hamilton Rating Scale and therefore it was not possible to verify a greater, more specific action in any single item. One of the more characteristic aspects of depression is represented by anxiety; however, in the present study this was difficult to evaluate in response to the treatment as the concomitant use of a benzodiazepine certainly modified the entity. Therefore, it cannot be suggested that Rubidium improves anxiety, but it is evident that, during treatment, this symptom was favourably modified by relatively low and constant doses of benzodiazepine.

The patients who improved with the treatment came from different diagnostic groups and, due to the limited number of patients it was not possible to draw secure conclusions on which type are better responders. However, it may be suuggested that both bipolar depressives and major depressives seem to respond positively to the treatment. Moreover, evaluation after the period of treatment has evidentiated that the effect of rubidium is long-lasting and that it is maintained even after withdrawal of the compound.

The side effects observed during treatment were only slight and therefore did not hinder the continuation of the study. This confirmed the excellent tolerance of the product at the doses and times studied. Neither did the laboratory tests evidentiate the appearance of abnormal features after the treatment, indicating a good level of tolerance of rubidium.

On the basis of these preliminary data and considering the results in literature on this matter, it would seem to be useful to further the study of this cation by means of controlled double-blind studies with placebo, in order to define the antidepressant spectrum of activity in a greater number of patients. Furthermore, a better definition of the kinetic aspects with an evaluation of the therapeutic blood levels would contribute towards a more rational and controlled use of the drug.

REFERENCES

1. Botkin S.S. : The influence of the salts of rubidium and cesium upon the heart and circulation in connection with the laws of physiological action of alkali metals. Doct.diss, St.Petersburg (1888).
2. Meltzer H.L., Taylor R.M., Platman S.R. and Fieve R.R.: Rubidium: A potential modifier of affect and behaviour. Nature 233, 321-322, 1969.
3. Stolk J.M., Nowack W.J. and Bargaas J.D.: Brain norepinephrine: enhanced turnover after rubidium treatment. Science 168, 501-503, 1970.
4. Colburn R., Goodwin F. and Bunney W.E.Jr: Effect of Lithium on the uptake of noradrenaline by synaptomsomes. Nature 215, 1395-1397, 1967.
5. Gessa G.L. Unpublished results. 1983.
6. Wang Y.C., Pandey G.N., Mendels J., Frazer A.: Effect of Lithium on prostaglandin E1 stimulated adenylate cyclase of human platelets. Biochem.Pharmacol. 4, 845, 1974.
7. Kupfer D.J., Wyatt R.G., Greenspan K., Snyder F.: Lithium carbonate and sleep in affective illness. Arch.Gen.Psychiat. 23, 261-268, 1970.
8. Maggini C., Andreoli V., Guazzelli M.: Studio poligrafico del sonno in maniaci ed ipomaniaci trattati con carbonato di litio. Riv.Neurol.45, 209-216, 1975.
9. Meltzer H.L., Lubermann K.W.: Chronic ingestion of rubidium without toxicity: implication for human therapy. Experientia 6, 672, 1971.
10.Meltzer H.L., Fieve R.R.: Rubidium in psychiatry and medicine: an overview. In: Essman W.B. and Valzelli L. (eds.), Current Developments in Psychopharmacology, pp.205-242, 1975.
11.Fieve R.R., Meltzer H.L., Taylor R.M.: Rubidium Chloride ingestion by volunteer subjects: initial experience. Psychopharmacologia 4, 307-316, 1971.
12.Fieve R.R., Meltzer H.L., Taylor R.M.: Rubidium: biochemical, behavioural and metabolic studies in humans. Am.J.Psychiat. 1, 55-61, 1971.
13.Carolei A., Sonsini V., Casacchia M., Agnoli A., Fazio C.: Azione farmacologica del cloruro di rubidio. Effetto antidepressivo: confronto con l'imipramina. Clin.Terap. 75, 469-478, 1975.
14.Chouinard G., Annable L.: The effect of Rubidium in schizophrenia. Commun. Psychopharmacol. 1, 373-383, 1977.
15.Chouinard G., Annable L.: Effect of Rubidium Chloride on the course of schizophrenia. New Research Abstract, 132nd Meet.of the Am.Psychiatric Ass. Chicago, 1979.
16.Paschalis C., Jenner F.A., Lee C.R.: Effects of Rubidium Chloride on the course of manic-depressive illness. J.Ray.Soc.Med.71, 343-352, 1978.
17.Calandra C., Nicolosi M.: Confronto fra due farmaci ad azione antidepressiva: Rubidio cloruro e clorimipramina. Proc.of 34th Cong.of Italian Society of Psychiatry, Catania, Italy, 1980.

19
The use of rubidium chloride in depressive disorders: clinical aspects

M. CASACCHIA, A. ROSSI, V. MAROLA AND G. MECO

INTRODUCTION.

Rubidium,discovered in 1861,by Bunsen and Kirchoff,is one of the Group
1 A alkali metals belonging to the same periodic series as lithium,so-
dium,potassium and cesium.It is widely distributed in mineral deposits
and can be extracted from lepiodolite and carnallite rocks,wich are also the major sources of lithium. Rubidium is also present in virtually
all biological systems.Physiologically,rubidium most resembles potassium,and these two elements have a great degree of metabolic interchange-
ability. Meltzer and his group(1) early reported that rubidium increased the prevalent frequency of the EEG in monkeys and altered the behavior in the direction of increasea activity. So it has been hypothesize
d that rubidium,like lithium,might therefore have application in psycho
pharmacology,particularly in the affective disorders.Moreover Stolk et
al.(2) suggested that rubidium enhanced the turnover of norepinephrine
in rats whose biosynthesis of norepinephrine was inhibited.Further observation of Stolk et al.(3) demonstred that rubidium increased normeta
nephrine formation in rat brain,an effect opposite to that seen with li
thium. In 1971 Fieve et al.(4) reported initial experience on RbCl ingestion by volunteers subjects:in that time the rediscovery of rubidiu
m was started. As lithium appears to be a specific "replacement-like"
therapy for mania,so it has been hypothesized that rubidium might offer
the same chance for one or more depressive disorders(5).In the last 10
years very few clinical experiences about rubidium effects are available in literature(6). Four manic-depressive patients were treated with
rubidium chloride therapy;two patients had a prolonged manic phase(7).
The purpose of this study is the assesment of the therapeutic effect
of rubidium in depressive patients in correlation with the plasma level of this substance and the monitoring of side effects.

METHODS

We carried out a comparison between Rubidium Chloride abd Imipramine
in single blind traatment.Depressed patients were selected who met
DSM III criteria for affective disorders(8) and who had been free of
psychotropic drugs other than benzodiazepines for at least three weeks.
Of 44 patients included in the treatment, 2 patients on rubidium did
not complete the period of treatment(1 discontinued for deterioration,
1 for intercurrent illness). In the Imipramine group two patients discontinued for adverse reactions. Of 40 patients, 20 were treated with
Imipramine (150 mg./daily) and 20 with rubidium chloride(540 mg./daily
in three doses). Both groups were similar in diagnosis,sex,age, lenght
ofillness and severity on admission.Before treatment and on days 7,14,
21,28 patients were assessed using the Hamilton rating scale for use
in depression(9). Demographic and diagnostic data are provided in table
1. Paired comparisons were made using Wilcoxon's signed Rank Test.Serum
level of rubidium was assessed at the end of treatment according with
Sutter et al.(10).

Table 1.

	RbCl	Imipramine
Number	20	20
Age —mean	52	51.5
—range	18–71	25–68
Sex —male	10	10
—female	10	10

Diagnosis
     —major depression
        single episode
	6	6

—major depression recurrent	10	9
—dysthymic disorder	4	5
Daily dosage	540 mg	150 mg

Results

Table 2 shows the therapeutic effect of two drugs over the time in HRSD
total score.Both drugs produced significant improvement from 7th onward.

Table 2. Results on the Hamilton Depression Rating Scale(HRS)

HRS	baseline mean±SE	day 7 mean±SE	day 14 mean±SE	day 21 mean±SE	day 28 mean±SE
IMI	28.5±0.7	22.0±1.1	17.9±1.1	14.5±1.1	13.5±1.2
RbCl	29.3±1.2	22.7±1.3	20.1±1.4	16.5±1.5	14.9±1.4

no significant differences were observed between paired values

There was a trend for Imipramine to be more effective than Rubidium but this difference was not statistically significant.At the end of both treatments the HRSD total score showed improvement "much" and "very much" in more than 50% of patients (Tab.3).

Table 3. Percent of patients with different improvement measured by HRS at the last assesment during RbCl and Imi treatment.

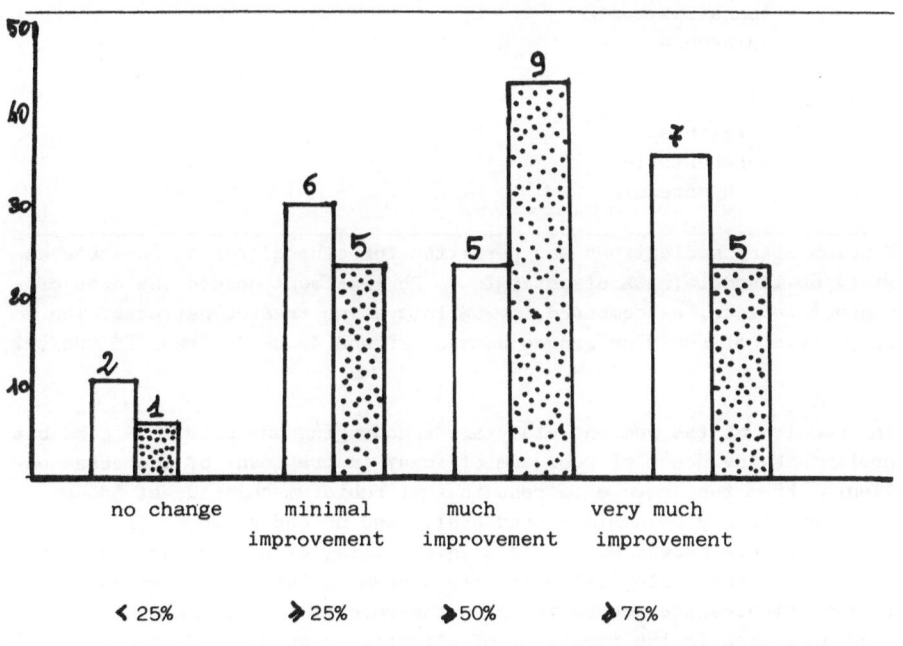

Side effects monitoring were obtained by direct questioning and spontaneous reporting (Tab.4). Imipramine treatment was often associated with autonomic side effects (dry mouth, constipation) or cardiovascular (orthostatic hypotension) side effects; rubidium treatment was more often associated with excitament.

Table 4. Percentage of patients reporting specific side effects.

effect	RbCl	Imipramine
Behavioral toxicity		
-agitation	10	0
-drowsiness	0	30
-insomnia	10	0
-fatigue	0	40
Neurologic		
-tremor	0	5
Autonomic		
-dry mouth	5	50
-constipation	5	40
-diarrhea	5	0
Cardiovascular		
-dizziness	0	30
-orthostatic hypotension	0	30

Supplementary medications was permitted for ethical reason in acute anxiety or insomnia; 30% of patients on Rb treatment needed one dose of benzodiazepines, as compared to 20% Imipramine treated patients. The serum level of rubidium ranged between 15 and 43 uEq/L (mean 25 uEq/L).

COMMENT

The results of the present study are encouraging and provide a good but preliminary evidence of rubidium efficacy in treatment of depressed patients. From the above data results that rubidium chloride at 540 mg daily can safely be administered orally and no undesirable clinical side effects are shown. However a clinical trial of a drug such rubidium, that has a long biological half-life present a lot of problem and so further studies are needed to value the role of rubidium and his mechanism of action in the treatment of affective disorders. Metabolic studies will be necessary to assess toxicity and tolerance level in humans.

REFERENCES

1) Meltzer,H.L.,Täylor,R.M., Platman,S.R. et al. (1969).Rubidium: a potential modifier of affect and behavior.Nature,233,321-22.

2) Stolk,J.M.,Conner,R.L.,Barchas,J.D.(1971).Rubidium-induced increase in shock elicited aggression in rat.Psycopharmacologia,22, 250-260.

3) Stolk,J.M.,Nowack,Barchas,J.D.,Platman,S.R.(1970).Brain norepinphrine:enhanced turnover after rubidium treatment.Science,168, 501-3.

4) Fieve,R.R.,Meltzer,H.L.,Taylor,R.M.(1971).Rubidium chloride Ingestion by volunteer subjects:initial experience.Psycopharmacologia,20,307-14.

5) Fieve,R.R.,Meltzer,H.L., et al.(1973).Rubidium:Biochemical, Behavioral,and metabolic studies in Humans.Am.J.Psychiatry,130,55-60.

6) Carolei,A.,Sonsini,U.,Casacchia,M.,Agnoli,A., Fazio,C.,(1975). Azione farmacologica del cloruro di rubidio.Effetto antidepressivo: confronto con l'imipramina.La Clinica Terapeutica,75,469-78.

7) Paschalis,C.,Jenner,F.A.,Lee,C.R.(1978)Effects of rubidium chloride on the course of manic-depressive illness.J.R.Soc.Med.71, 343-352.

8) American Psychiatric Association,Committee on Nomenclature and Statistics.(1980)Diagnostic and Statistical Manual of Mental Disorders,ed.3.Washington,D.C.,American Psychiatric Association.

9)Hamilton,M.(1967).Development of a rating scale for primary depressive illness. British Journal of Social and Clinical Psycology, 6,278-96.

10)Sutter,E.,Platman,S.R.,Fieve.R.R.(1970).Atomic absorption spectrophotometry of rubidium in biological fluids. Clin.Chem.,16,602.

Part V
New Aspects in
Lithium and
Rubidium Treatment

20
The effect of lithium treatment in humans of psychophysiological increases and decreases in heart rate

S. CHAZAN-GOLOGORSKY, P. GOLAN, S. KUGELMASS AND R. H. BELMAKER

INTRODUCTION

Two psychophysiological heart rate response phenomena have been noted
and investigated in the literature: heart rate acceleration and heart
rate deceleration. These two responses of the cardiovascular system
have been associated with cognitive functioning and orienting response
situations, respectively. In the 1950's, it was believed that increased
sympathetic activity had an excitory and facilitating effect, serving
to provoke or maintain cortical activation. Lacey (1) observed that
this did not hold for increases in heart rate and blood pressure. He
claimed that heart rate increase would most likely be coupled with a
reduced sensitivity to stimulation. Lacey proposed that heart rate
increase should be associated with lowered sensitivity to the environment and should occur in situations of painful or unpleasant stimulation,
or in situations where external distractions would interfere with
internal problem-solving. Conversely, Lacey postulated that heart rate
decrease should be associated with heightened sensitivity to stimulation and should occur in a situation requiring "attention". These
proposals were confirmed by Obrist (2). Cardiac changes were also seen
by Sokolov (3) to be under the control of environmental inputs. He
considered these changes to be a component of the orienting response,
defined as a functional system which enhances sensitivity to external
stimuli. Sokolov did not discuss the significance of the direction of
cardiac change. However, on the basis of Lacey's work, deceleration

263

would be expected.

Lacey (4) reported a correspondence between heart rate deceleration and stabilization during attentive observation of the external environment. This author is well known for his empirical design which consisted of flashing nude figures on a screen observed by male subjects who displayed heart rate deceleration in anticipation of the stimuli. Porges and Raskin (5) supported Lacey's finding and in their own research demonstrated that heart rate variability was sensitive to attentional demands. They claimed that subjects involved in attentional tasks responded with significant reductions in heart rate. Rogers, Bankart and Light (6) also reported partial confirmation of their prediction that heart rate would fall in anticipation of shock.

In 1970, Obrist evaluated two hypotheses related to the association between performance on a simple reaction time task and heart rate deceleration. Two groups were tested. In one group, the cardiac response was blocked pharmacologically in order to determine if this response facilitated performance through an afferent feedback mechanism. They found that blocking the cardiac response did not significantly influence task performance. However, within-subjects analysis revealed a direct relationship between reaction time and the magnitude of cardiac deceleration when the latter was not blocked pharmacologically.

In 1972, Porges designed an experiment investigating the differential relationship among heart rate variability, deceleration and attentional performance during a reaction time task. Subjects were required to perform one of two tasks: a. Respond as quickly as possible following the termination of an extended visual warning signal, or b. To merely observe non-signal visual stimuli. He found that following the onset of the warning signal, heart rate variability increased and decreased in anticipation of signal termination. This suggests a possible biphasic response pattern which has been widely discussed in the literature, but shall not be dealt with in the present paper.

Belmaker et al (7) applied Lacey's theory regarding heart rate acceleration to the investigation of the effects of lithium on the cardiovascular system and heart rate reactivity. They hypothesized that "lithium in vivo is a physiological inhibitor of noradrenergic function, perhaps in the brain as well as the heart". Furthermore, they predicted that the effect on the biochemical level would be reflected on the psychophysiological level, i.e. heart rate activity. In clinical studies, Tilkian et al (8) reported that lithium has some antiarrhythmic effect in man. Belmaker et al (7) compared the performance of manic-depressive patients receiving lithium to that of normal drug-free controls on mental arithmetic tasks. They found that lithium-treated subjects displayed consistantly smaller heart rate increases with each task as compared to those shown by the controls. They also found that the effect of lithium was only on the cardioacceleratory response and not on baseline heart rate, which did not show any reduction. They theorized that lithium may block heart rate activation without affecting baseline activity. Furthermore, actual performance on mathematical tasks did not seem to be hampered by lithium, as no significant difference on this dimension was found between the two groups.

Table 1. Heart Rate Increases[a] During Mental Arithmetic Tasks in 22 Lithium-Treated and 17 Untreated Subjects

Task	Lithium Group		Untreated Group		Significance[b]
	Mean	SEM	Mean	SEM	
Counting backward	3.5	1.7	7.4	1.7	p=.07
Addition problems	6.8	1.0	12.9	1.7	p<.05
Multiplication problems	7.3	1.2	12.8	1.8	p<.05
Reverse spelling	4.4	.7	11.2	1.8	p<.05

[a] In beats per minute over mean resting heart rate (lithium group=78.4 ±2.4 SEM; untreated group=80.7±2.9 SEM; difference is not significant).

[b] One-tailed Student's t test

(From Belmaker et al, 1979)

Reactivity may be examined on both the physiological and the psychological-behavioral levels. One may investigate responses elicited by any change of stimuli occurring in the motor, autonomic or central nervous systems. The orienting response, for example, has been defined as "a system of unconditional...responses elicited by any change in stimulation independent of stimulus quality" [Sokolov, (3)]. Thus heat and cold would evoke an orienting response when first presented although upon repetition each would evoke a distinct adaptation reaction. One problem of the studies relating to the orienting response is that they lack the information necessary to identify the response. For example, when a response is averaged across trials it is difficult to ascertain whether there was habituation or intensification with stimulus repetition.

On the behavioral level, it has been found that individuals respond to different stimulus situations in their own unique ways. That is, "for a given set of autonomic functions, individuals tend to respond with a pattern of autonomic activation in which maximum activation will be shown by the same physiological function" [Wenger, (9)]. People who react with elevated heart rates to stress situations, will tend to react with the same physiological responses across similar situations. This phenomenon is known as response specificity.

In the present study, physiological reactions are measured while the implications are considered at the psychological level. Our assumption is that absolute changes of heart rate are a physiological manifestation of the subjects' interpretation of, and reaction to, the experimental situation.

The rationale behind the present study is based on our previous research [Belmaker et al, (7)] in which we found that there was a differential reactivity of lithium patients and normal subjects to an experimental stimulus. The paradigm presented by Belmaker et al (7), was designed to evoke heart rate increases. We hypothesize that a similar trend, in an opposite direction, will be found when subjects are exposed to a situation which is believed to bring about heart rate decelerations. That is to say, lithium patients will show less reactivity, i.e. smaller decreases in heart rate, than will normal controls.

METHODS
Subjects

Subjects consisted of two groups: 19 euthymic manic-depressive patients attending a lithium clinic where they are maintained on a controlled lithium program and 18 drug-free control subjects randomly selected from the staff of Ezrath Nashim Psychiatric Hospital. The ages of both groups ranged between 25 and 75. The average age of the lithium experimental group was 46.3 and for the control group 41.4.

Apparatus

I. A Tachometer with a recorder and finger monitor attachment was used to measure heart rate patterns.

II. A stimulus panel box was designed which consisted of a set of two lights, one red and one green. Below the lights was a response button, which when pressed, switched off the red light. The lights were timed so that when the start button was pressed, the green light would light up for 10 seconds after which the red light would reappear for a maximum duration of 5 seconds. Following this period, both lights would extinguish for a resting period of 30 seconds. At the termination of 30 seconds, the green light would reappear and the sequence would be repeated.

Procedure

Subjects were identified and seated in a small room adjoining a laboratory in which the heart rate machine was placed. They were told to relax and then were given a brief introduction to the experiment and instructions concerning their task:

We are interested in seeing the time it takes for people to respond to stimuli. Before you, there is a box with two lights: one green light and one red one. At some point after the start of the exercise, a green light will appear. At this point, keep your eyes on the light and await the appearance of the RED light. When this light appears, press on the button directly below it and this will turn off the light. Please do this as quickly as you can. After this light goes off, you may relax. This is the end of the first exercise. The next trial will begin again with the appearance of the green light. At this point, you will begin once again.

Following these instructions, a finger monitor was placed on the thumb on the non-dominant hand. Subjects were told to relax so that a base-

line could be measured. When the heart rate recorder showed
relatively stable beats, a one minute baseline measure was taken. At
the end of one minute, the experiment commenced. Four trials were
recorded and the total procedure was of 6-10 minute duration for each
subject.

Analysis of Data

Baseline was calculated by averaging the heart rate measures at
intervals of 5 seconds over a 40 second period. Heart rate decreases
were computed during the 10 second trials by taking the greatest difference between the highest and lowest heart rate measures where these
appear consecutively, following the first two seconds of stimulus onset.
Heart rate decreases were averaged over the four trials.

A statistical analysis of data was made using multiple analysis of
variance. Age and baseline were covaried due to the disparity of the
averages between experimental and control groups.

Table 2. Heart Rate Decreases (beats per minute) in an Attention
Paradigm for 19 Lithium-Treated and 18 Control Subjects

	Lithium-treated		Controls		Univariate significance
	Mean	SEM	Mean	SEM	
Baseline heart rate	81.0	3.2	86.8	3.2	t=1.27 p=.21 ns
Age	46.3	2.5	41.4	3.3	t=1.18 p=.25 ns
Heart rate decrease	2.64	.46	5.52	.92	After simultaneous covariance for age & baseline HR, decrease in HR is significantly different F=5.3 p=.02

RESULTS

The average decrease in heart beats per minute for lithium-treated
patients was $2.64 \pm .46$ (SEM) and for controls $5.52 \pm .92$. This difference
in heart rate decrease between lithium-treated and control groups was
significant in a univariate test, Student's t =2.75, p < .02.   Age and

baseline heart rate were not significantly different between the groups
in a univariate test. Co-variance with HR was computed for age and baseline variables separately. Only age was found to be a significant
covariant of HR deceleration scores. The significance of t for age as
a covariant with HR deceleration was p=.013 and for baseline HR as a
covariant of HR deceleration, p=.296. Simultaneous covariance of age
and baseline heart rate before comparing heart rate decreases in the
two groups revealed a significant difference after covariance, F=5.3
p=.02

DISCUSSION

In the present study, it was found that heart rate deceleration was
significantly smaller for lithium-treated patients than for drug-free
controls. This finding may be discussed on both the physiological and
the psychological levels.

Previous research findings suggest that lithium may affect the cardiovascular system by inhibiting noradrenergic adenylate cyclase and thus
inhibiting the function of the sympathetic nerves to the heart [Belmaker
et al (7)]. The question arises regarding the extent of lithium's
effect on the autonomic nervous system (ANS). That is, does the drug
have a generalized effect on all aspects of the ANS or is it specific to
cardiovascular activity? If lithium has a generalized effect,
differences in ANS activity would be found between lithium-treated and
control groups across all areas of the ANS. Galvanic skin response (GSR)
is presently being examined in an attempt to explore this question.

Another possibility is that subjects may respond individually to
stimuli (external or internal). If lithium has a generalized effect on
the ANS, it may be manifested differentially in accordance with
individual response specificity. For example, some people may respond
to stimuli with heightened cardiovascular activation, while others may
tend to do so with greater GSR. It would be interesting to examine
whether lithium's possible generalized effect might in particular lower
reactivity in that specific area of the ANS in which the individual
tends to respond. Example: If Individual A responds to stress
predominantly with heightened cardiovascular activity, would lithium's
effect then be mainly localized in this part of the ANS rather than in
other areas?

We may interpret our findings of smaller heart rate deceleration in lithium-treated patients in terms of a lowered reactivity to stimulus situations. Lithium patients showed no significant reduction in baseline heart rate. Significant differences between groups were found only in the magnitude of their reaction to stimuli. Therefore, while heart rate baseline averages do not appear to be affected by lithium, reactivity seems to be lowered. This is consistant with Belmaker et al (7) in which we found that resting baseline HR and performance on mathematical tasks were not affected by lithium, while heart rate increases during the mental tasks were reduced. The baseline heart rate of control subjects was nonsignificantly higher in the present experiment, whereas no such trend was evident in the previous study [Belmaker et al, (7)]. This may be due to the fact that baseline measures were taken just prior to the experiment onset in the present study, whereas a habituation period was included in the previous study. Since lithium patients were familiar with the laboratory surroundings, the absence of a habituation period may have affected their baseline heart rate less than that of hospital employee volunteers, who were new to the role of experimental subject.

The James Lange-theory of emotion suggests that peripheral arousal contributes to the brain's perception of emotion. If lithium tends to lower reactivity to outer stimuli, then the lithium patient may perceive himself as being less aroused. Dampened affect arousal may in turn affect cardiac responsivity, and lowered heart rate may again cause perception of lowered arousal. Thus a feedback system may be established between autonomic response and the individual's psychological assessment of his inner state.

It was not possible for us in the present study to include either a "normal" lithium-treated group or a lithium-free manic-depressive group. Thus one cannot differentiate between the effect of the illness and that of lithium on cardiovascular reactivity. It is possible that manic-depressive patients are less reactive in HR than controls and that this is unrelated to lithium.

Some methodological problems of the present study should be noted: a. No measure was taken of the speed at which subjects responded to the stimulus. Therefore, it is not possible to discuss lithium's effect on task performance; b. Deceleration measures were averaged over four trials. Thus, the means obtained do not take into account the possibility of adaptation to stimuli or fatigue factors. Lang and Hnatiow (10) found that although acceleration remained constant across trials, deceleration decreased with stimulus repetition. In the present study, four trials were used for reliability purposes. It would, however, be possible to examine each trial separately and to study adaptability trends. If habituation is a factor, then our findings represent a more conservative estimate of the deceleration phenomenon, as adaptation would cause diminishing reactivity over trials for both groups; c. Deceleration may be influenced by a breathing artifact, particularly in the case of younger subjects. That is, deceleratory responses may be due in part to the effect of breathing on heart rate and not to stimulus response.

Conclusion

Our findings seem symmetrical to those previously found by Belmaker et al (7), where lithium-treated patients tend to show lower heart rate increases to mental arithmetic. These preliminary studies seem to suggest a generalized effect of lithium on the ANS. It would be interesting to determine whether the phenomenon of lower reactivity is found across all areas of the ANS by examining pupil dilatory responses, GSR, etc.

REFERENCES

1. Lacey, J.I. and Lacey, B.C. (1958). The relationship of resting autonomic activity to motor impulsivity. In: The Brain and Human Behavior. (Baltimore: Williams, Wilkins)

2. Obrist, P.A. (1963). Cardiovascular differentiation of sensory stimuli. Psychosom. Med., 25, 450-459

3. Sokolov, E.N. (1960). Neuronal models and the orienting reflex. In: Braxier, M.A.B. (ed). The Central Nervous System and Behavior. pp.187-276. (New York: Macy Jr. Foundation)

4. Lacey, J.I. (1967). Somatic response patterning and stress: some revisions of activation theory. In: Appley, M.H., Trumball, R. (eds). Psychological Stress: Issues in Research. (Appleton-Century-Crofts)

5. Porges, S.W. and Raskin, D.C. (1969). Respiratory and heart rate components of attention. J. Experimental Psych., 81, 497-503

6. Rogers, W., Bankart, B., Light, J. (1970). Differences in the motivational significance of heart rate and palmar conductance: two tests of a hypothesis. J. Personality & Soc. Psych., 14(2), 166-172

7. Belmaker, R.H., Lerner, R., Ebstein, R.P., Lettik, H., Kugelmass, S. (1979). A possible cardiovascular effect of lithium. Am. J. Psychiatry, 136:4B, 577-579

8. Tilkian, A.G., Schroeder, J.S. et al. (1976). Cardiovascular effects of lithium in man: a review of the literature. Am. J. Medicine, 61, 665-670

9. Wenger, M.A., Clemens, T.L., Coleman, D.R. et al. (1961). Autonomic response specificity. Psychosom. Med., 23, 186-193

10. Lang, Hnatiow. (1962). Stimulus repetition and heart rate response. J. Comp. and Physio. Psych., 55, 781-785

21
Left ventricular performance following lithium treatment

M. R. PISANO, R. FONZO, M. DEL ZOMPO, P. BONOMO, G. U. CORSINI AND A. CHERCHI

INTRODUCTION

Since the original discovery of the antimanic properties of lithium in 1949 (1), a large number of studies have confirmed the efficacy of this drug in the treatment of mania (2), as prophylactic agent in unipolar and bipolar affective illness (3-5) and as antidepressant drug (6). Furthermore, the usefulness of lithium has been evaluated in various other psychiatric and non-psychiatric illnesses (7). It is generally considered that therapeutic doses of lithium do not adversely affect cardiac function (8,9); nevertheless, there are numerous reports concerning the effects of lithium on the heart.

The most frequent electrocardiographic changes consist of T-wave flattening or inversion (8-15). Other cardiac effects of lithium therapy are observed more rarely, such as atrial (16-26) and ventricular arrythmias (8,27), conduction disturbances and cardiomyopathies (20,28,29,30).

All these reports suggest that, although clinical experience attests to the safety of lithium therapy, therapeutic levels of lithium have been associated

TABLE I   CLINICAL DATA

Pt	Sex	Age (years)	Psychiatric diagnosis	Phisical Findings	Lithiaemia mean values (mEq/l)	Other drugs
1	F	53	MD	N	0.81	Sulpiride 50 mg/die
2	F	65	BDI	N	0.54	Amitryptiline 50 mg/die
3	F	35	BDI	N	0.69	Levomepromazine 25 mg/die
4	F	70	BDII	N	0.63	
5	M	62	MD	HBP	0.59	Chlorpromazine 50 mg/die
6	F	59	MD	N	0.65	Mianserine 20 mg/die
7	F	78	BDI	N	1.15	Thioridazine 75 mg/die
8	F	54	SD	SM	0.68	
9	F	69	BDII	SM	0.65	Amitryptiline 10 mg/die
10	F	59	BDII	N	0.84	
11	F	72	SD	SM	0.90	Levopromazine 50 mg/die
12	M	49	BDI	N	0.80	Chlorpromazine 200 mg/die
13	F	67	BDI	SM,HBP	0.69	Chlorpromazine 50 mg/die
14	F	32	BDII	SM,HBP	0.65	Chlorimipramine 45 mg/die
15	F	56	BDI	HBP	0.81	
16	F	48	MD	N	0.65	
17	F	41	SD	HBP	0.62	
18	M	58	SD	N	0.80	
19	F	70	BDI	AI	1.04	
20	M	62	BDI	N	0.96	

Abbreviations: N = normals; SD = schizoaffective disorders; BDI = bipolar disorders I;
BDII = bipolar disorders II; MD = major depression; SM = sistolic murmur;
AI = aortic insufficiency; HBP = high blood pressure.

with cardiac disfunction. Furthermore, there have been few studies to evaluate
the effects of therapeutic doses of lithium in psychiatric patients, not only
on the electrocardiogram (ECG) but, more importantly, on myocardial function
(31,32). Thus, we studied the effects of therapeutic doses of lithium on
left ventricular performance in twenty psychiatric patients who had been under
lithium therapy for more than three years.

METHODS

Twenty patients, 4 men and 16 women, aged between 32 and 78 years, suffering
from various psychiatric disorders (33) were studied (Table 1).

Patients were studied only after informed consent had been obtained from
them concerning all procedures. The patients were visited periodically in the
Lithium Clinic of Clinical Pharmacology, University of Cagliari.

All the patients had been undergoing long-term treatment with lithium
carbonate for at least three years, some of them following other therapy
concurrently (Table 1). The patients received lithium carbonate in a range of
dosage between 300mg and 1200mg per day and their mean lithiaemia was approximately 0.70 ± 0.159 mEq/l.

They underwent clinical evaluation, M-mode ecocardiography and phonocardiogram. The clinical examination included a family history and physical exam,
with special attention given to the cardiovascular examination. The phonocardiogram was carried out in fasting patients after five minutes rest in
supine position using an OTE BIOMEDICA polianalyser 1126 with paper speed of
100mm/sec.

TABLE II   M-MODE ECHOCARDIOGRAPHIC VALUES DURING LITHIUM THERAPY

Pt	AO mm	LA mm	EF mm/sec	EDD mm	EDS mm	ΓS %	PWTh mm	PWFT %	IVSTh mm	IVSFT %
1	21	33	51	37	24	34	9	34	8	47
2	36	36	56	48	27	44	12	33	12	44
3	27	35	65	50	30	39	7	101	7	67
4	25	37	59	43	26	38	6	82	6	66
5	35	39	48	52	29	43	7	81	8	82
6	32	44	79	59	37	36	9	56	8	66
7	24	40	104	68	47	31	8	66	8	66
8	33	40	40	52	28	46	8	66	8	66
9	32	33	80	47	33	29	7	61	8	50
10	28	35	40	51	32	37	9	70	9	70
11	35	32	67	52	33	32	9	56	9	72
12	32	40	29	47	28	39	7	101	13	30
13	25	40	102	55	35	36	7	60	7	101
14	31	44	81	49	33	32	11	50	11	37
15	31	51	55	57	35	39	9	43	7	101
16	28	29	64	48	32	33	7	82	8	50
17	28	41	64	57	33	41	9	56	9	72
18	33	47	78	53	37	30	11	50	9	56

Abbreviations: AO = aortic dimension;LA = left atrium dimension; EF = mitral
valve E-F slope;EDD = left ventricular end-diastolic dimension;EDS = left ventricular end-systolic dimension;FS = left ventricular fractional shortening;
PWTh = left ventricular posterior wall thickness;PWFT = left ventricular posterior wall fractional thickening;IVSTh = interventricular septum thickness;
IVSFT = interventricular septum fractional thickening.

Systolic time intervals were measured using the method of Weissler et al. (34). Each interval was calculated taking the average of at least four consecutive measurements. The M-mode Echocardiogram was carried out in eighteen of the twenty patients, after five minutes rest in a supine position, in fasting conditions, using an echocardiovisor 3 of Organon Teknika, with a 2.25 MHz transducer, collimated to 7.5cm. M-mode tracings and an ECG were recorded on a Honeywell LS-6A strip-chart recorder at a speed of 50mm/sec. The dimensions of the aortic root and left atrium, mitral EF segment slope, telediastolic and telesystolic left ventricular dimensions, fractional shortening, telediastolic thickness of the interventricular septum and of the posterior wall of the left ventricle with their respective percentages of thickening were calculated. The various parameters were calculated according to the directions of the European Society of Cardiology (35).

The values obtained in our patients were compared with the normal values of Roelandt (36). The echo and phonocardiograms were repeated in five patients who had an above normal PEP/LVET ratio fifteen days after withdrawal of the drug.

RESULTS

Clinical Data (Table 1).

The clinical examination demonstrated a mild systolic ejection murmur in five patients and blood pressure values above normal in five patients; one patient presented a murmur of aortic regurgitation.

Echocardiographic data (Table II).

The dimension of the aorta was found to be normal in all eighteen of the patients in whom it was possible to perform an echocardiogram. The dimensions of the left atrium were found to be increased in five patients; the slope

TABLE III   SYSTOLIC INTERVAL TIMES DURING LITHIUM THERAPY

Pt	$Q-S_2I$	LVETI	PEPI	ICT	$Q-S_1I$	PEP/LVET
1	531	414	116.7	37	56.5	0.2908
2	516	386	129	35	58	0.3856
3	552	429.2	122.8	40	58	0.2969
4	525	407	118	24	60	0.2491
5	536.5	399.5	137	35	68	0.4039
6	557	422	133.2	51	61	0.3313
7	532	405.6	126.4	35	65	0.3333
8	558	442	116	28	60	0.2666
9	529	381.8	147.2	57	63	0.4395
10	550	401.8	148.2	38	77	0.4275
11	542	384.4	157.6	64	70	0.4620
12	525.7	412.9	112.8	33	75	0.2943
13	536	427.2	108.8	36	49	0.2560
14	562	410.1	158.4	49	75	0.4200
15	569	440.4	128.6	50	61	0.3000
16	552	417	135	66	47	0.3434
17	546	394.8	151.2	50	70	0.4444
18	563	424	139	27	80	0.3715
19	576	455	121.1	33.5	68	0.2695
20	560.8	440.6	120.2	25	68	0.3793

of the echocardiographic mitral EF segment resulted decreased in relation to the normal values of Roelandt (76mm/sec.) in II cases. The diastolic dimensions of the left ventricle were shown to be above the normal maximum values in 4 cases. The fractional shortening, the thickness of the posterior wall of the left ventricle and of the interventricular septum and the percentage of systolic thickening was found to be normal in all the patients examined with the exception of the one patient who had mild septal hypertrophy (13mm).

Systolic Time Intervals (Table III).

The PEP/LVET ratio was above the maximal normal value in seven patients.

Echocardiographic data after lithium withdrawal (Fig.1.).

Echocardiograms performed following the withdrawal of lithium do not show any significant changes with respect to those performed during administration of the drug.

Systolic Time Intervals after Lithium withdrawal (Fig.2.).

A decrease in the PEP/LVET ratio was observed from the phonocardiograms carried out following withdrawal of lithium (from 0.43 ± 0.01 to 0.39 ± 0.03) without this difference being statistically significant, while the decrease in QS_1 following withdrawal of the drug appeared to be significant (from 69.6 ± 5.0 to 61 ± 8.8 msec) ($p < 0.05$).

DISCUSSION

Analyzing our results, it is of importance to note the absence of cardiovascular symptoms even though five patients presented blood pressure values above normal, and one patient presented aortic insufficiency of little hemodynamic importance. The echocardiogram showed atrial enlargement in approximately one-third of the patients and ventricular dilatation in about one-quarter of them.

The thickness of the left ventricular wall (posterior wall and interventricular septum) was found to be normal in all patients, except one who had a septum with an increased thickness. The most frequently altered data in the echocardiogram was the EF segment slope, reduced

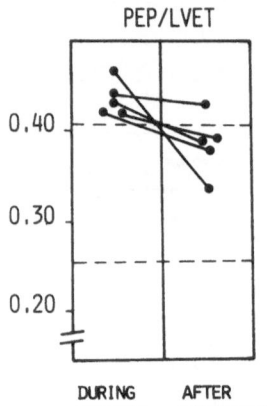

PEP/LVET

0.40

0.30

0.20

DURING   AFTER
LITHIUM   WITHDRAWAL

FIGURE 1 DURING LITHIUM THERAPY FIVE CASES SHOWED AN INCREASE OF PEP/LVET RATIO. FEFTEEN DAYS AFTER LITHIUM WITHDRAWAL FOUR OF THEM WERE FOUND IN NORMAL RANGE.

in 61% of the cases. In the absence of mitral stenosis, this reduction is to be attributed to either a decreased elasticity of the mitral leaves or to a decrea sed ventricular compliance due to sclerosis and thickening found in elderly subjects (37). The left ventricular fractional shortening and the systolic thickening percentage of the posterior wall and of the septum were within nor- mal limits in all cases.

This suggests that ventricular function in these patients treated with lith- ium, regarded both as global and regional ventricular function, was normal. An analysis of systolic time intervals demonstrated the PEP/LVET ratio, one of the most expressive, non invasive, parameters of left ventricular func- tion, to be increased above normal in 35% of the patients. Contrary to previous ly examined echocardiographic data, this analysis showed an alteration of an important index of left ventricular function in seven patients.

In an attempt to demonstrate the influence of lithium on alteration of the above mentioned parameter, we suspended the drug in five of the seven patients. It was not possible to discontinue the drug in the other two due to their pre- carious mental conditions. These five patients underwent an echocardiographic and phonocardiographic re-examination 15 days after drug withdrawal. The re- sults of the echocardiogram following suspension of lithium (Fig.2) demonstra- te that the withdrawal of the drug does not determine a significant variation of the different parameters.

The results of the phonocardiogram following drug withdrawal (Fig.1.) sho- wed a non significant decrease in PEP/LVET ratio (from 0.43 ± 0.01 to 0.39 ± 0.03). It is important to note that in four patients the ratio decreased substantially, returning to the range of normal values, while in one patient af- fected with arterial hypertension and treated with diuretics, sus- pension of the lithium brought about only a slight decrease.

Non significant variations were also found with regard to QS_2, PEP and LVET. In particular, PEP decreased (from 148 ± 7.4 to 142 ± 6.0 msec), without reaching statistical importance.

To further examine the behaviour of PEP, the two frac- tions that make it up were calculated: the electromechanical latency (QS_1) and the isovolu- metric contraction period (ICT), both evaluated as M1 carotid rise time and calculated, in our case, as S_1S_2-LVET. Of these above mentioned elements, the former is

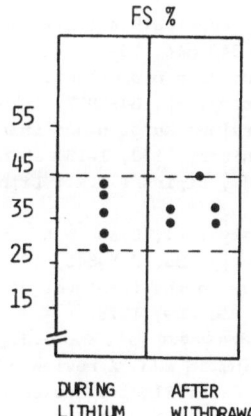

FIGURE 2   THE FIVE CASES WITH INCREASE OF PEP/LVET RATIO (FIG.1) SHOWED NORMAL VALUES OF FRACTIONAL SHORTENING DURING AND AFTER LITHIUM WITHDRAWAL.

related to the conduction velocity of the cardiac muscle fibers. The latter is related to the pressure rise velocity within the left ventricle from enddiasto-lic ventricular pressure values to those of aortic diastolic pressure. The Ml-carotid rise time represents only a part of the isovolumetric contraction pe-riod, as the mitral valve closes after the beginning of ICT; since we are con-cerned with comparisons in which the individual patient is his own control, this method is valid to evaluate the variation in duration of ICT.

The isovolumetric cotraction time did not result as being significantly modified following drug withdrawal, while QS_1 is significantly reduced from 69.6 $\pm$5.0 msec to 61 $\pm$ 8.8msec (p < 0.02). This reduction of QS_1 observed fol-lowing the discontinuation of lithium is probably due to an increase in con-duction velocity in the specific conduction system. As a matter of fact, it is known that the administration of lithium salts causes a modification of the membrane potential, with a decrease in both the resting membrane potential and the velocity of the rise of the action potential, with a consequent de-crease of the fiber conduction velocity (20).

In conclusion, based on our results, we can state that the long term administration of lithium salts, at therapeutic doses, does not have a negative influence on left ventricular function, as shown by the normal values for global and regional ventricular function in the echocardiogram.

The alterations of systolic time intervals observed in a few of the patients demonstrated a tendency to decrease following drug withdrawal, probably due to an increase of the conduction time, reduced in lithium therapy.

REFERENCES

1. Cade J.F.: Lithium salts in the treatment of psychotic excitement. Med.J.Aust., 2, 349-352, 1949.
2. Goodwin F.K., Athanasios P.Z.: Lithium in the treatment of mania. Arch.Gen. Psychiatry, 36, 840-844, 1979.
3. Schou M.: Lithium as a prophylactic agent in unipolar affective illness. Arch.Gen.Psychiatry, 36, 849-853, 1979.
4. Davis J.M.: Overview: Maintenance therapy in psychiatry. II Affective Disor ders. Am.J.Psychiatry, 133, 1-13, 1976.
5. Baldessarini R.J., Lipinski J.F.: Lithium salts: 1970-1975. Intern.Med. 83 527-533, 1975.
6. Mendels J., Ramsey T.A., Dyson W.L. et al.: Lithium as an antidepressant. Arch.Gen.Psychiatry, 36, 845-846, 1979.
7. Schou M.: Lithium in the treatment of other psychiatric disorders. Arch.Gen Psychiatry, 36, 856-859, 1979.
8. Tilkian A.G., Schoroeder J.S, Kao J.J., Hultgren H.N.: The cardiovascular effects of lithium in man. A review of literature. Am.J.Med.61,665-670,1976
9. Wren J.C., Dana J.B.: Electrocardiographic changes during lithium therapy. J.Maine Med.Ass.6, 185-189, 1976.
10. Andreani G.: Electrocardiographic findings during treatment with lithium salts. J.Clin.Med. 38, 1759-1775, 1957.
11. Demers R.G., Heninger G.R.: Electrocardiographic T-wave changes during li-thium carbonate treatment. Div.Nerv.Syst.31, 674-679, 1970.
12. Demers R.G., Heninger G.R.: Electrocardiographic T-wave changes during li-thium carbonate treatment. J.Am.Med.Ass. 218, 381-386, 1971.

13. Hansen H.E., Amdisen A.: Lithium intoxication (report of 23 cases and review of 100 cases from the literature). Quart.J.Med.47, 123-144, 1978.

14. Kochar M.S., Wang R.I.H., D'Cunha G.F.: Electrocardiographic changes stimulating hypokaliemia during treatment with lithium carbonate. J.Electrocardiol., 4, 371-373, 1971.

15. Schou M.: Electrocardiographic changes during treatment with lithium and with drugs of the imipramine-type. Acta Psychiatr.Scand. 38, 331-336, 1962.

16. Eliasen P., Andreani M.: Sinoatrial block during lithium treatment. Eur.J. Cardiol., 3, 97-98, 1975.

17. Wellens H.J., Cats V.M., Duren D.R.: Symptomatic sinus node abnormalities following lithium carbonate therapy. Am.J.Med. 59, 285-287, 1975.

18. Wilson J.R., Kraus E.S., Bailas M.M., et al : Reversible sinus node abnormalities due to lithium carbonate therapy. New Eng.J.Med.294, 1223-1224, 1976.

19. Roose S.P., Nurnberger J.I., Dunner D.L., Blood D.K., Fieve R.R.: Cardiac sinus node disfunction during lithium treatment. Am.J.Psychiatry, 136, 804-806, 1979.

20. Riciutti M.A., Lisi K.R., Damato A.N.: A metabolic basis for the electro physiological effects of lithium. Circulation (suppl.II) 44-45: 217, 1971.

21. Humbert G., Fillastre J.P., Leroy J., Maitrot B., Tobelem G., Leroux G., Lavoine A.: Intoxication par le lithium. Sem.Hop.Paris, 50, 509, 1974.

22. Schou M., Amdisen A., Trap-Jansen J.: Lithium poisoning. Am.J.Psychiatr., 125, 520-524, 1968.

23. Constans R., Chapelet A., Marco J., Dardenne P.: Observation cliniques-clinical records "Dysfonctionnement sinusal reversible au cours d'un traitment par le carbonate de lithium". Acta Cardiologica T. XXXIII, 5, 315-322, 1978

24. Le Heuzey J.Y., Degusseau B., Belliard J.P., Soulie J., Grivaux M: Dysfonctionnement sinusal troubles de conduction etages et intoxication par le lithium. Sem.Hop.Paris 54, 303-305, 1978.

25. Hagman A., Arnman K., Ryden L.: Syncope caused by lithium treatment. Acta Med.Scand. 205, 467-471, 1979.

26. Morena H., Denis B., Chaltiel G., Jacquot C., Machecourt J., Martin-Noel P: Coeur et lithium. Arch.Mal.Coeur, 70, 741-748, 1977.

27. Tangedahl T.N., Gau G. T : Myocardial irritability associated with lithium carbonate therapy. New Engl.J.Med.287, 867, 1972.

28. Kleinert M.: Myocardiopathie untar lithium therapie. Med.Klin.69, 494, -499, 1974.

29. Tseng H. Interstitial myocarditis probably related to lithium carbonate intoxication. Arch.Pathol. Lab.Med. 92, 444-448, 1971.

30. Swedberg K., Winblad B.: Heart failure as a complication of lithium treatment. Acta Med.Scand.196, 279-280, 1974.

31. Dumovic P., Burrows G.D., Chamberlain K., Vohra J., Fuller J., Sloman J.G.: Effect of therapeutic dosage of lithium on the heart. Br.J.Clin.Pharmac. 9, 599-604, 1980.

32. Tilkian A.G., Schroeder J.S., Kao J .J., Hultgren H.: Effect of lithium on cardiovascular performance: report on extended ambulatory monitoring and exercise testing before and during lithium therapy. Am.J.Cardiol. 38, 701-708, 1976.

33. Spitzer R.L., Endicott J., Robins E.: Research Diagnosis Criteria (RDC) for a selected group of functional disorders, Third.Ed. New York State Psychiatric Institute, Biometrics Research, 1977.

34. Weissler A.M., Harris W.J., Schoenfeld C.D.: Bedside technics for the evaluation of ventricular function in man. Am.J.Cardiol. 23, 577, 1969.

35. Gruppo di lavoro ecocardiografico della Società Europea di Cardiologia. Raccomandazioni per la standardizzazione delle misure sugli ecocardiogrammi M-mode. G.Ital.Cardiol. 9, 920, 1879.

36. Roelandt J.: Normal ecocardiographic values. In: Practical Echocardiology, Vol.One, pp.283, Research Studies Press, 1977.

37. Fonzo R., Sau F., Seguro C., Mercuro G., Lai C., Cioglia G., Cherchi A. : Valori ecocardiografici normali: influenza dell'età. In corso di stampa. Rass.Med.Sarda 1982.

22
Lithium carbonate and granulocyte function during cancer chemotherapy. Preliminary report

S. MILANI, G. MUSTACCHI, F. DE LAZZER, P. SANDRI, S. DE LUYK, C. PICCININI, N. FERRRANTELLI, L. LINDA AND E. RORAI

INTRODUCTION

Lithium has recently been used in association with cancer chemotherapy(CT). Granulocytic leukopenia is one of the major side effects of CT; it leads to the risk of serious infections and to antineoplastic drug doses reduction, preventing a correct therapeutic schedule. Therefore lithium, that induces a reversible neutrophilia, probably increasing colony stimulating factor(I) and peripheral PMN survival(2), has been promoted as an adjuvant in CT (3). There are many data about effectivness of lithium in attenuating leukopenia and neutropenia, but there is little information about PMN function during lithium treatment. If the increase of PMN count is accompanied by a reduction of their functional capacity, lithium treatment would be of little usefulness. There is some controversy on this subject and only very few studies are dealing with cancer patients(4). In a previous study(5), we too demonstrated the positive effect of lithium on WBC count and PMN count during antiblastic treatment. Now we want to test a possible effect of lithium on PMN function, in cancer patients undergoing CT.

MATERIALS AND METHODS

Patients population. 20 women with breast cancer, developing
leukopenia(i.e.: WBC count less than 4000 per cu mm) during
CT(CMF or AV protocols) were randomly allocated to receive
lithium carbonate, 300 mg orally 3 times a day for 7 days
or placebo. No other drug was administered during this period. IO women, age ranging from 36 yrs to 74 yrs, mean age
of 54.7 yrs, entered the lithium group; IO women, age ranging from 35 yrs to 74 yrs, mean age of 53.8 yrs, entered
the control group.

Laboratory tests. At leukopenia time(To) and after 7 days
(Tl), WBC count, PMN count, PMN phagocytic activity were
performed.

Phagocytic activity test. We used the method outlined by
P. Bellavite and Coll.(6), based on the quantitative measurement of superoxide anion(O_2^-) produced by PMN_s.
0.2 ml of venous blood, mixed with a solution of preser-
vative-free heparin, IO U/ml, were added to zimosan, I mg,
and cytocrome C, 3 mg, diluted in 0.8 ml of KRP buffer, and
incubated in a 37°C water bath for I5 min. 4 ml of KRP, at
4°C, were added; the sample was centrifugated at 2000 g for
IO min. The test was repeated adding 0.02 ml of SOD(2.5 mg
per ml). The difference between the O.D. of the 2 samples
supernatants was determined, obtaining the O_2^- nmoles produced by the PMN_s. The results were expressed per IO^6 PMN_s and
per cu mm of blood.

Statistical evaluation. The two-tailed Student's t test was
used.

RESULTS

WBC count. Lithium group, starting from a mean value of 3I90
+/- 530 at To, reached a Tl mean value of 48IO +/- I7IO with
a difference statistically significant(s.s.-p < 0.02).
Control group: the To mean value was 3095 +/- 608; the Tl
mean value was 3869 +/- II50, with no significant difference
(n.s.).

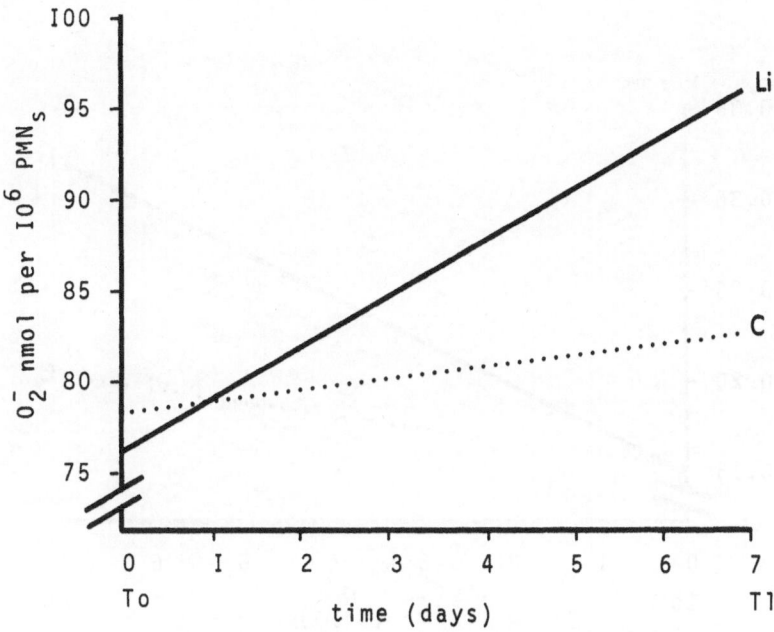

FIGURE I Effect of lithium on PMN phagocytosis during cancer chemotherapy. Mean values expressed as O_2^- n-
moles produced by 10^6 PMN$_s$.

PMN count.Lithium group: the initial mean value was 1978 +/-
590. After 7 days treatment the mean value was 3224 +/-1178
(s.s.-p<0.01). Control group starting from a To mean value
of 1985+/-570, reached a T1 mean value of 2546+/-1009(n.s.).
Phagocytic activity. (O_2^- nmoles per 10^6PMN$_s$- Fig.I). Lithium group: the functional capacity showed an increase, however not significant, from the before treatment mean value
of 76.2+/-27.4 to a T1 mean value of 95.6+/-32.1.
Control group: To mean value of 78.3+/-18.1 changed up to
T1 mean value of 82.7+/-21.2(n.s.).
Phagocytic activity. (O_2^- nmoles per cu mm blood- Fig.2).
Lithium group: To mean value of 0.15+/-0.06; T1 mean va-
lue of 0.32+/-0.19 with an evident positive trend .
Control group: from To mean value of 0.16+/-0.05 reached a
T1 mean value of 0.20+/-0.07(n.s.).

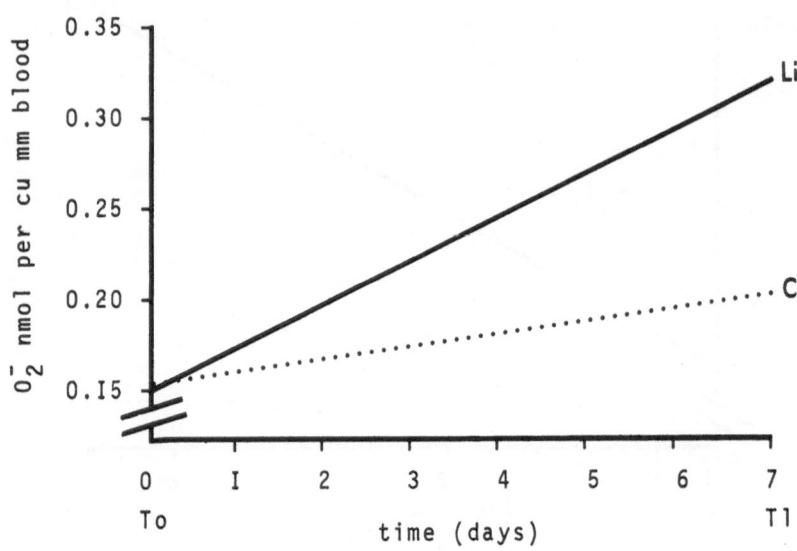

FIGURE 2 Effect of lithium on PMN phagocytosis during cancer chemotherapy. Mean values expressed as O_2^- n-
moles produced per cu mm of blood.

For each parameter considered, there was no significant
difference between the lithium group To and the control group To mean values. Comparing the lithium group T1 and the
control group T1 mean values, we found a positive trend in
favour of the lithium group in the WBC and PMN counts.
Only mild gastrointestinal side effect was noted in 2 lithium patients.

DISCUSSION

Lithium has been introduced in cancer therapy to offset the
leukopenia and neutropenia induced by antineoplastic drugs.
To assess a real usefulness of the lithium treatment, it is
important to evaluate not only number but even functional
capacity of PMN_s. It was also reported that PMN functions
are generally depressed in cancer patient, with or without
chemotherapy(7). In vivo studies concerning random migration,

chemotaxis, phagocytosis and bactericidal ability reported normal, depressed or enhanced activities after lithium treatment(4). Very few studies concern cancer patients.

For each test performed, we found in the lithium treated group an increase between before and after treatment values. The statistical significance of the variation of WBC and PMN counts confirms previous data. It is expecially noteworthy the enhancement of the phagocytic activity. It was important not to find a decrease in the functional PMN capacity after lithium. In the lithium patients, we noted a positive trend- a difference statistically not significant, however interesting-in the PMN function. It is not fully understood by which mechanism lithium can affect this function: cyclic nucleotides are supposed to play an important role in modulating many cells activity and it may be that lithium effect is mediated by inhibiting adenylate ciclase activity(8).

The test we used to assay the PMN phagocytic function gives some advantages as compared to other methods: it requires a very little blood amount, is very quick and relatively simple to perform and has a very good sensitivity.

Our study is still ongoing and these are some interim results, regarding only a little number of cases. However these preliminary data are encouraging and the positive trend in the lithium treated patients indicates a possible effect of lithium in increasing not only PMN number, but even PMN activity.

REFERENCES

I.   Richman, C.M., Kinnealey, A. and Hoffman, P.C. (I98I). Granulopoietic effect of lithium on human bone marrow in vitro. Exp. Haematol. 9, 448-55

2.   Rothstein, G., Clarkson, D.R., Larsen, W., Groner, B.I. and Athens, J.W. (1978). Effect of lithium on neutrophil mass and production. N. Engl. J. Med. 26, I78-80

3. Lyman, G.H., Williams, C. and Preston, D. (1980).
The use of lithium carbonate to reduce infection and leukopenia during systemic chemotherapy. N. Engl. J. Med. 302,
257-60

4. Friedenberg, W.R. and Marx,J.J. (1980). The effect of
lithium carbonate on lymphocyte, granulocyte and platelet
function. Cancer 45, 91-7

5. Mustacchi, G., Milone, E., Ginanneschi, U. and Milani,
S. (1982). Effect of lithium carbonate on leukopenia induced by antimethabolic drug in rats. Rec. Med. XXI, 176-84

6. Bellavite, P., Dri, P., Berton, G. and Zabucchi, G.
(1980). A new method based on measurement of anion superoxide production to test phagocytic function. Lab. VII,
67-76

7. Garelli, S., Valbonesi, M., Schieppati, G. and Banfi,
L. (1981). Defective function of granulocytes in patients
with cancer. Tumori 67, 415-25

8. Shenkman, C., Borkowsky, W., Helzman, R.S. and Shopsin, B. (1978). Enhancement of lymphocyte and macrophage
function in vitro by lithium cloride. Clin. Immunol. Immu-
nopathol. 10, 187-92

23
Cancer chemotherapy induced neutropenia: effects of lithium carbonate

E. T. MENICHETTI, R. R. SILVA AND R. CELLERINO

INTRODUCTION

It is well known that Lithium Carbonate, which is utilized
in psychiatric patients, induces a reversible neutrophilic
leucocytosis which persists during the administration and
resolves within a week of discontinuance of the drug (7-8).
During cancer chemotherapy, neutropenia is one of the most
frequent and harmful side-effects because of the possibili
ty of infectious events and the necessity of reducing drug
dosage and/or delaying the performance of therapeutic cour
ses, compromising treatment efficacy (1).
In this study we evaluated the ability of Lithium to affect
the neutropenia associated with cancer chemotherapy and its
real clinical role.

METHODS

We studied 25 patients affected by solid tumors in different evolutive phases and treated with antiblastic chemotherapy. All patients before entering the study had already received at least three chemotherapeutic courses.

287

Patients under the age of 70, with Karnofsky Performance Status higher than 50 and life expectancy exceeding 6 months were admitted to the study. Patients with haematolo gical neoplasias and those undergoing treatment with steroids were excluded.

Patients entering the study were randomized into two groups: 11 patients received Lithium Carbonate 300 mg three times a day by mouth for 14 days before each therapeutic course (300 mg twice a day were administered to patients with body area less than 1.5 square meters). This dosage allowed to maintain Lithium serum levels between 0.7 and 1.4 mEq/liter.

The remainig 14 patients formed the control group.

Of the 11 patients admitted to the Lithium group, 2 patients were afterwards not able to be evaluated: one because Lithium had been discontinued, the other because he had been treated with no more than three courses.

Of the 14 patients admitted to the control group, 3 were not able to be evaluated because they had been treated with no more than three courses.

Characteristics of the patients, which are comparable in the two groups, are reported in table 1.

Therapeutic schedules foresaw intervals of 21-28 days between one course and the other and utilized a combination of 2-3 drugs. The drugs used are summarized in table 2. There is no statistically significant difference between the two groups.

Red blood cell count, haemoglobin dosage, total and differential white blood cell count and platelet count were done before each therapeutic course; percentage of drug do sage and time employed for the administration of therapeutic courses in comparison with theoretical standards were measured; incidence of infectious events was recorded.

RESULTS

In table 3 and 4 and in figure 1 are reported mean values
of peripheral leucocytes and neutrophils.
In table 5 and 6 are reported mean values of platelets and
of haemoglobin dosage.
Mean values of circulating leucocytes do not show statisti
cally significant defferences between the two groups.
On the contrary mean values of neutrophils show a statisti
cally significant difference, in favour of the Lithium
group, at the 3rd ($p<0.05$) and 4th ($p<0.02$) chemotherapeutic course.
We did not observe any statistically significant difference between the Lithium group and the control group with
regard to the platelet count and haemoglobin dosage.
The antiblastic drug amount effectively administered in per
cent of the theoretical dosage is reported in table 7.
Even if there is an advantage for the Lithium group the
difference is not statistically significant; besides which
the dosage used in each group is very close to the theoretical one.
With regard to the time employed for the performance of
therapeutic courses, we measured the weeks lost due to neu
tropenia in comparison with the theoretical time; mean per
cent values show that the control group had a statistically significant delay (table 8).
No infectious event occurred in either group of patients.
The side effects reported by patients receiving Lithium
were a slight tremor of the hands in 2 cases and a mild
weakness in 1 case. These effects did not result in a dis

continuance of Lithium therapy.

DISCUSSION

The most important principles in applying cancer chemotherapy are the respect of the proper dosing and of the inter
vals of administration (1-4-9).

Our study seems to indicate a clear advantage in favour of
the Lithium group because of a major regularity in the
administration of therapeutic courses without long delays
due to neutropenia.

These observations confirm the experience of others (6).
Our impression however is that the effect on neutrophils
is time-limited (2-3 months): this fact may represent a
progressive decrease of the stem-cell potentiality as observed by others (2).

Lithium seems to be ineffective on platelets and on haemoglobin according with the observations of other Authors
(6-11).

The mechanism of Lithium-induced neutrophilia is still under discussion.

Studies on murine bone marrow in culture reported an activity of Lithium on the grouth of CFUc (Colony Forming Unit
in culture) (5-12). This activity is likely due to an increase of the production of CSF (Colony Stimulating Factor) by competent cells (5).

This effect, confirmed by studies on humane bone marrow in
culture (10), is probably mediated by inhibition of cAMP
system (3).

Table 1. Characteristics of the patients

	Controls (N 11)	(%)	Lithium (N 9)	(%)
Median age	42 50 62		36 57 69	
M/F	3/8		2/7	
Breast ca.	2	(18)	4	(44)
Gastric ca.	3	(27)	3	(33)
Melanoma	4	(36)	1	(11)
Colo-rectal ca.	1	(9)	1	(11)
Ovarian ca.	1	(9)	/	/
Advanced disease	5	(45)	3	(33)
Bone metastases	4	(36)	2	(22)

Table 2. Drugs

	Controls	(%)	Lithium	(%)
Adriamycin	4	(36)	4	(44)
5-Fluorouracil	7	(64)	7	(78)
Mitomycin-C	3	(27)	3	(33)
Carmustine	2	(18)	1	(11)
Ciclophosphamide	3	(27)	3	(33)
Dacarbazine	4	(36)	1	(11)
Methotrexate	2	(18)	3	(33)
Vincristine	1	(9)	1	(11)

Table 3. Peripheral leucocyte count: mean values ± standard deviation   (leucocytes/mm^3)

	Controls	(N)	Lithium	(N)	
1st course	6436 ± 2490	(11)	2922 ± 1932	(9)	NS
2nd "	4600 ± 1723	(11)	5288 ± 1315	(9)	"
3rd "	4372 ± 1247	(11)	5566 ± 1379	(9)	"
4th "	4950 ± 2674	(11)	4933 ± 1979	(9)	"
5th "	4950 ± 2674	(10)	4962 ± 1510	(8)	"
6th "	4600 ± 1308	(8)	4583 ± 1993	(6)	"

Table 4. Peripheral neutrophil count: mean values ±standard deviation   (neutrophils/mm^3)

	Controls	(N)	Lithium	(N)	
1st course	3936 ± 1618	(11)	3155 ± 891	(9)	NS
2nd "	2690 ± 956	(11)	2811 ± 1040	(9)	"
3rd "	2418 ± 842	(11)	3388 ± 645	(9)	p<0.05
4th "	2381 ± 1170	(11)	4133 ± 1656	(9)	p<0.02
5th "	3310 ± 2299	(10)	2722 ± 746	(8)	NS
6th "	2875 ± 1296	(8)	3100 ± 1253	(6)	"

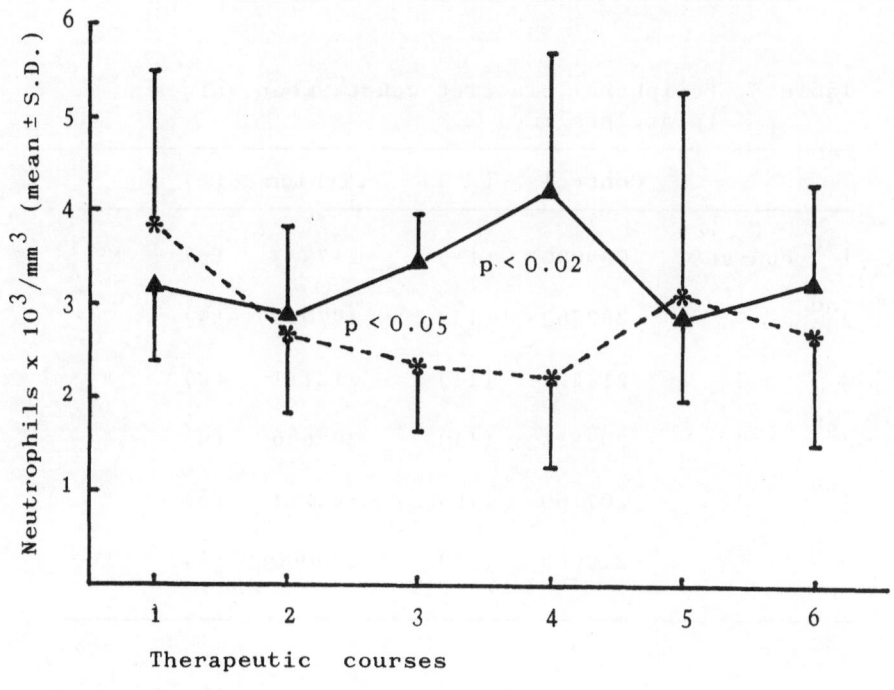

Figure 1: Graphic representation of neutrophils trend.

Table 5. Peripheral platelet count: mean values
          (platelets/mm^3)

		Controls	(N)	Lithium	(N)	
1st	course	239090	(11)	217333	(9)	NS
2nd	"	262363	(11)	197000	(9)	"
3rd	"	215272	(11)	2121II	(9)	"
4th	"	203545	(11)	202666	(9)	"
5th	"	207100	(10)	194111	(8)	"
6th	"	219666	(8)	228000	(6)	"

Table 6. Haemoglobin dosage: mean values ± standard
          deviation   (g/100 ml)

		Controls	(N)	Lithium	(N)	
1st	course	12.5 ± 1.5	(11)	12.5 ± 1.9	(9)	NS
2nd	"	12.4 ± 1.4	(11)	12.1 ± 2.0	(9)	"
3rd	"	12.2 ± 1.4	(11)	12.2 ± 2.0	(9)	"
4th	"	11.8 ± 2.1	(11)	11.5 ± 3.1	(9)	"
5th	"	11.7 ± 1.3	(10)	11.7 ± 2.5	(8)	"
6th	"	12.3 ± 1.5	(8)	12.0 ± 2.8	(6)	"

Table 7. Drug dosage: mean percent values ± standard
deviation

		Controls	(N)	Lithium	(N)	
1st	course	93.18 ± 16.16	(11)	94.44 ± 11.02	(9)	NS
2nd	"	90.90 ± 20.22	(11)	94.44 ± 11.02	(9)	"
3rd	"	93.63 ± 15.66	(11)	97.22 ± 8.33	(9)	"
4th	"	95.44 ± 15.05	(11)	94.44 ± 11.02	(9)	"
5th	"	92.05 ± 16.87	(10)	96.87 ± 8.83	(8)	"
6th	"	90.00 ± 19.27	(8)	100.00 ± 0.00	(6)	"

Table 8. Percent of weeks lost due to neutropenia: mean
percent values ± standard deviation

		Controls	(N)	Lithium	(N)	
1st	course	0	(11)	0	(9)	
2nd	"	3.03 ± 10.04	(11)	3.70 ± 11.11	(9)	NS
3rd	"	8.32 ± 12.35	(11)	1.85 ± 5.55	(9)	"
4th	"	9.59 ± 9.00	(11)	1.23 ± 3.70	(9)	$p < 0.02$
5th	"	13.27 ± 12.32	(10)	2.07 ± 5.86	(8)	$p < 0.05$
6th	"	11.51 ± 10.44	(8)	1.66 ± 2.58	(6)	$p < 0.05$

REFERENCES

1) Bonadonna, G., Valagussa, P. (1981). Dose-response effect of adjuvant chemotherapy in breast cancer.
New Engl. J. Med., 304, 10-15

2) Casirola, G., Invernizzi, R., Ippoliti, G. et al. (1980)
Effetti del Litio carbonato sulle neutropenie primitive e secondarie. Haematologica, 65, 746-754

3) Chan, H, S. L., Saunders, E.F., Freedman M.H. (1980).
Modulation of human hematopoiesis by prostagladins and Lithium. J. Lab. Clin. Med., 95, 125-132

4) De Vita, V.Jr, Hellman,S., Rosenberg,S. (1982).
Cancer: principles and practice of Oncology pp. 140-141
(J.B. Lippincott Co. Philadelphia, Toronto).

5) Harker, G.W., Rothstein, G., Clarkson, D. et al. (1977).
Enhancement of colony-stimulating activity production by Lithium. Blood , 49, 263-267

6) Lyman, G.H., Williams,C.C., Preston,D. (1980). The use of Lithium carbonate to reduce infection and leukopenia during systemic chemotherapy. New Engl. J. Med., 302, 257-260

7) Radomsky, J.L., Fuyat, H.N., Nelson, A.A. et al (1950).
The toxic effects,excretion and distribution of Lithium chloride. J. Pharmacol. Exp. Ther., 100, 429-444

8) Risetto, G., Gassano, G. (1952). Variazione del sangue periferico nella intossicazione sperimentale da sali di Litio. Riv. Patol. Clin. Sper.,7 202-205

9) Schabel,F.M.Jr, Simpson- Herren, L. (1978). Some variables in experimental tumor systems which complicate interpretation of data from in vivo kinetic and pharmacologic studies with anticancer drugs. Antiblastic Chemotherapy, 23, 113-127

10) Spitzer, G., Verma, D.S., Barlogie, B. et al. (1979).
Possible mechanisms of action of Lithium on an augmenta-
tion of in vitro spontaneus myeloid colony formation.
Cancer Res., 39, 3215-3219

11) Stein, R.S. (1977). Lithium carbonate in chemothera-
py-induced neutropenia. New Engl. J. Med., 297, 1180

12) Trivisonne, R., Piga, A., Cellerino,R. (1981). Effetto del Litio sul midollo emopoietico murino coltiva-
to in vitro. Tumori, 67, suppl.2 , 171

24
Lithium and rubidium compounds in cluster headache: overview and perspectives

F. SAVOLDI, G. BONO, G. C. MANZONI, G. MICIELI, M. LANFRANCHI AND G. NAPPI

Among the various forms constituting the spectrum of headache disorders
cluster headache (CH) certainly is the most peculiar and represents an
interesting model of dysrhythmic condition involving nociception, endocrine and autonomic symptoms. The most common variety of the disease,
episodic CH, displays a circannual pattern similar to peptic ulcer and
cyclic depression, but also in the chronic type the typical circadian
and ultradian occurrence of the attacks is observable (1,2). The pathogenesis of CH is still unknown and an involvement of CNS has been proposed, based on the alterations found in several rhythmic biological
functions as well as on the effects of some drugs and procedures able
to interfere with the course of periodic disorders of central origin
(3,4,5).

Ten years have passed since the introduction of Lithium salts in CH
prophylaxis and, despite the agreement on its effectiveness (6,7), some
questions remain to be settled concerning in particular the outcome of
long-term treated patients, the ability to interfere with the natural
history of the disease and the perspectives for the Lithium tolerant
cases of chronic CH. The aim of the present paper is to discuss the
results of Lithium salts effects and to suggest the prophylactic use
of other compounds (rubidium salts) in this disease. Preliminary to

these topics, a few details will be given about the clinical feature and some problems related to CH pathogenesis.

CLUSTER HEADACHE

(a) Clinical aspects. The term "cluster headache" gained widespread use following the observations of Ekbom and Kunkle (8,9), who described the typical cyclical pattern of the circannual periods of the disease (cluster periods) and the circadian timing of the attacks (cluster attacks). The particular grouping of the headache attacks usually defines one or two active periods a year, each lasting 6-12 weeks and usually occurring during times of change, such as of the seasons or of lifestyle linked, for example, to new work schedules. Contrary to views previously held, single cluster attacks only rarely present a characteristic autumn-spring course: detailed study has shown that, with the exception of a biphasic summer pattern, variations in the frequency of the headache periods are associated with changes in atmospheric temperature. Remission phases, lasting from a few months to many years, separate the cluster attacks. The occurrence of attacks during a 24 hour period also follows a cyclical pattern, appearing one or more times for thirty minutes to two hours. The main entraining factors are represented by the sleep-wake cycle and mealtime schedule, or, more generally, by any series of events, internal or external, which constitute a fixed time program of activity. Moreover, the attacks are concentrated with clock -like regularity in the very late night hours, in the early afternoon (often after lunch) or after the evening meal (10).

The term cluster headache is the one most in favour among the workers in the field; however, this condition is also known by other terms, of which the most commonly used are histamine headache and Horton's headache. Besides, there is a whole series of names derived from the attempt to define cluster headache in terms of neuronal pathways or on the basis of autonomic manifestations accompanying the pain (11). However, in spite of its use in literature, the term "cluster" headache remains

unsatisfactory. In fact, chronic forms of cluster "sine cluster" exist
in which the periodic clustering of the attacks is absent, sometimes
from the very beginning. This pattern is characterized by the absence
of remissions for at least one year, by a progressive increase in the
frequency of attacks and by a decreased response to prophylactic therapy. The chronic form can be such right from the start or appear after
a period of time, years or even decades, of a typical episodic pattern.
In most cases there is no particular problem in making the differential
diagnosis from other primary and symptomatic headaches. Pain distribution in CH follows a rigid topographic pattern (behind and around the
eye with subsequent radiation to the temporal, frontal and facial
areas). In addition, there is a marked increase in motor activity:
patients cannot remain seated, become agitated, aggressive and at times
may even harbour thoughts of suicide. During CH attacks transient autonomic phenomena occur: tearing, red eye, partial "Horner", rhynorrea.
These signs always appear ipsilateral to the pain side and are generally reversible (12).

b) Pathogenetic considerations. Among the possible mechanisms which had
been invoked from time to time to explain the appearance of local autonomic signs during cluster attacks, the so-called central hypothesis
postulates that a primary alteration of CNS integrative mechanism,
probably at the hypothalamic level, is the decisive factor underlying
the autonomic phenomena (13). The hypothalamus is also the central sta-
tion of the limbic circuits, the true supervisor of the continuous flow
of primary sensory stimuli and at this level, emotional life is integrated with motor, endocrine and autonomic activities. At hypothalamic
level the rhythmic oscillations wich control adaptive functions to
external and internal environment are generated; there is also evidence
that these circuits intervene in the processes of modulation of physiological, right/left asymmetry, and, as is known, amplification of this
functional asymmetry may be the basis of disturbances involving mood,
sleep and nociception (14). Considering the picture of CH attacks,

neither parasympathetic hyperactivity nor sympathetic hypofunction can account, by themselves, for the whole series of signs and symptoms accompanying pain and the hypothesis of an unstable shifting between sympathetic and parasympathetic activity implying the involvement of central structures is also supported by neurophysiological and clinical-pharmacological evidences (15,16,17). On the other hand, the alterations found in several rhythmic biological functions related to body adaptive responses (5,18) point out a vulnerability of CNS oscillators and suggest the presence of a time structure alteration widely affecting neurotransmitters and neuro-hormones in different areas (limbic system; brain stem; striatum). On these alterations is based the so-called dyschronical hypothesis for CH. This is also supported by the effects of short-term sleep deprivation on the attack frequency and the circadian cortical pattern, as well as by the therapeutic effects of Lithium (5). Positive effects of sleep deprivation have been observed in depressed patients (3) and further investigations on circadian parameters will probably help clarify Lithium effects in CH as well as in other periodic disorders.

CLUSTER HEADACHE PROPHYLAXIS

a) Lithium compounds. Since the early reports by Ekbom, Graham and Rogado, several authors have evaluated the effects of Lithium in CH using different compounds: slow release sulphate preparations, Lithium orotate and carbonate (see Manzoni et al., Cephalalgia 1983, for a review). Studies conducted so far in the chronic form of the disease generally agree on the high effectiveness of Lithium therapy; less favourable results have been obtained in the episodic forms (19). In most of these investigations, however, the number of patients treated has been rather small.

An extensive analysis of the short- and long-term effects of Lithium treatment in CH has been recently reported by our group, concerning both episodic and chronic forms (7). The study included 90 patients under observation at the Pavia and Parma Headache Centres between 1977 and 1982. Their distribution by clinical subtypes and sex was as follows:

CH patients: 90 (78 M,12 F)

Episodic 68 (59 M,9 F)

Chronic   22 (19 M,3 F)

Primary 16 (14M, 2F)

Secondary 6(5 M, 1F)

Patients with chronic CH were followed for 3 to 48 months (average 22); in episodic CH the treatment was started on average 24 days (min 3, max 80) after the onset of a cluster period, 14/68 having been treated for more than one period. Lithium carbonate was employed at daily doses of 600 to 1200 mg (mostly 900 mg); Lithium levels were regularly monitored and the clinical improvement was quantified according to the Headache Index Ratio (10).

In the second week of Lithium treatment over 80% of the patients with chronic CH improved by more than 90%, and only 2 patients improved by less than 60%. The weekly HI of the 22 patients, which averaged 32.8 (min 12, max 65) prior to treatment, dropped to an average of 6.0 (min 0, max 24). In 7 patients side-effects did appear (tremor 4, diarrhoea 2, abdominal pain 1, olfactory hallucination 1, insomnia 1, vertigo 1, increased thirst 1) but they were mild and did not require drug discontinuation at this initial stage of treatment.

Later one, in the 4 patients who initially had improved by less than 90%, cluster attacks were still frequent or would frequently re-appear so that Lithium was discontinued after 3 to 6 months. The other 18 patients, who were followed for 9 to 48 months (average 27), exhibited two different patterns. In 11 patients the definite improvement observed soon after treatment start was almost unchanged; the other group (7 patients) worsened periodically, although the initial benefits deriving from treatment were still quite apparent in general (> 90%). No signifi_ cant differences were found in the distribution of patients with the primary or secondary form of headache between the groups with or without long-term benefits.

Plasma and erythrocyte Lithium levels varied from 0.3 to 0.8 meq/l and from 0.10 to 0.35 meq/l, respectively.

Among thr long-term side-effects, goitre developed in two cases (a 26-year-old woman in the 18th month of treatment and a 31-year-old man in the 40th month of treatment). This, however, did not impair the normal functioning of the thyroid gland and completely disappeared after Lithium discontinuation.

The effect of one or more interruptions of treatment on the CH course was evaluated in 9 patients. Two of them were the ones who had developed goitre. In the remaining seven cases, treatment was interrupted on purpose after 5 to 42 months in order to assess the resulting effects. In most cases (6 patients), the attacks re-appeared almost immediately, their frequency and intensity being sometimes higher than prior to treatment. All these patients, however, improved again dramatically when Lithium administration was resumed. In 3 patients, one with primary and two with secondary chronic CH, long periods of remission (6,4 and 8 months, respectively) were observed after treatment interruption, as if their chronic form had turned episodic.

Of the 68 patients with episodic CH, about three-fourths improved by more than 60%. In these patients (68) the weekly HI, which averaged 30.3 (min 12, max 58) prior to treatment, dropped to an average of 9.6 (min 0, max 42). Side-effects appeared in 18 cases, though in a mild form and not requiring treatment discontinuation; the most frequent among them were tremor, thirst and insomnia. Of the 16 patients who improved by less than 60%, 13 had Lithium discontinued before their cluster period was over because the drug had proved ineffective. In the remaining 55 patients, the cluster period on average lasted 43 days, which means that it was not significantly shorter than the average previous period (48 days). In no case did interruption of the treatment after the patients had been free from attacks for at least one week coincide with a re-appearance of the cluster period. The plasma and erythrocyte Lithium levels varied from 0.3 to 0.7 meq/l and from 0.12 to 0.34 meq/l, respectively.

When administered only within a cluster period, Lithium turned out to have no effect at all on the CH course. Fourteen patients were treated over two subsequent periods; in 3 of them the drug was considerably less effective in the second period than it had been in the first, whereas the remaining 11 patients improved as much in the second period as in the first. Four subjects with episodic CH were treated with Lithium carbonate without interruption for over a year: 3 cases because of the high frequency of cluster periods, and 1 case because the patient was also suffering from manic-depressive illness. In none of these 4 patients did attacks occur again as long as treatment was continued.

b) Rubidium compounds. Biochemical, behavioural and neuropsychological data (20,21,22) have pointed out the psychopharmacological properties of Rubidium and concurred to outline for this substance a profile which is "opposite" to that of Lithium. However, in some clinical studies Rubidium salts have proved effective in the treatment of depressed and schizophrenic patients (23,24). In the light of these observations we suggested to try this substance in CH, particularly in those patients suffering from very severe forms completely unresponsive or having become tolerant to Lithium.

Only 3 cases have been treated so far, but the results seem favourable and further observation is in progress. The patients were males, aged 34 and 45 yrs respectively, and had been suffering from 3 to 10 years from secondary chronic CH. They had previously undergone Lithium, methisergide, prednisone and ergotamine treatments, with variable responses, but no result could be obtained during the 3 months preceding Rubidium administration. The patients received doses of 180 mg Rubidium chloride three times a day for 8 weeks with accurate control of clinical effects and electrolite levels. No significant side-effect was reported while the 2nd week Headache Index resulted improved between

60 and 90% in two cases and almost unchanged in one.

One of the improved patients, in particular, who presented a base-line frequency of 3 to 6 attacks a day, only showed, at the 15th day control, the persistence of a single attack, regularly occurring after one hour of night sleep. Also this attack completely disappeared after administration of Nitrozepam (30 mg) at bed-time, being the patient symptom free during the 4 following weeks.

COMMENT

The analysis of our results points to some considerations. Lithium treatment is highly effective not only in short- but also in the long-term treatment of chronic CH, especially in those cases showing an over 90% short-term improvement; the daily doses are, on the average, slightly lower than those effective in the treatment of manic-depres-sive psychosis; Lithium is generally well tolerated even for long-term treatment; in some cases, fairly long periods of remission are observed after Lithium discontinuation; Rubidium treatment can be attempted in chronic CH patients who become tolerant to Lithium administration.

The mechanisms of action of Lithium and Rubidium in CH still remain to be explained. Lithium is known to influence sleep patterns as well as circadian systems (5) and these properties are in agreement with the evidences supporting the dyschronic hypothesis of CH (4). On the other hand, Lithium is known to reduce asymmetry in serotonin at the meso-limbic and mesostriated levels (14) and these effects have been corre-lated with the autonomic changes observed at the pupil level in CH patients after prolonged Lithium administration (Fanciullacci et al., present volume). Further chronobiological, biochemical and pharmaco-logical studies, however, are required for investigating Lithium and Rubidium effects on CH, an uncommon paradigm of cyclical and unilateral involvement of nociceptive and autonomic functions.

REFERENCES

1. Ekbom, K.L. (1979). Patterns of cluster headache with a note to the

relations to angina pectoris and peptic ulcer. Acta Neurol. Scand., 46, 225-37.

2. Dexter, J.D. and Weizman, E.D. (1970). The relationship of noctur-
    nal headaches to sleep stage patterns. Neurology, 20, 513-18.

3. Gerner, R.H., Post, R.M., Gillin, J.C. and Bunney, W.E. (1979). Bio
    logical and behavioral effects of one night's sleep deprivation in
    depressed patients and normals. J. Psychiat. Res., 15, 21-40.

4. Nappi, G., Micieli, G., Sandrini, G., Martignoni, E., Lottici, P.
    and Bono, G. (1982). Headache temporal patterns: towards a chrono-
    biological model. In: Nappi, G. and Sjaastad, O. (eds). Chronobio-
    logical Correlates of Headache, pp. 21-30.

5. Ferrari, E., Canepari, C., Bossolo P.A., Vailati, A., Martignoni,
    E., Micieli, G. and Nappi, G. (1982). Changes of biological rhythms
    in primary headache syndromes. Ibidem, pp. 58-68.

6. Kudrow, L. (1977). Lithium prophylaxis for chronic cluster head-
    ache. Headache, 17, 15-18.

7. Manzoni, G.C., Bono, G., Lanfranchi, M., Micieli, G., Terzano, M.G.,
    and Nappi, G. (1983). Lithium carbonate in cluster headache: assess
    ment of its short- and long-term therapeutic efficacy. Cephalalgia,
    3, 109-14.

8. Ekbom, R.A. (1947). Ergotamine tartrate orally in Harton's "Hista-
    minic Cephalalgia" (also called Harris "Ciliary Neuralgia"). Acta
    Psychiat., 46, 106-13.

9. Kunkle, C.E., Pfeiffer, J.B. Jr., Wilhoit, W.M. and Hamrick, L.W.
    Jr. (1952). Recurrent brief headache in "cluster" patterns. Trans.
    Amer. Neurol. Assoc., 77, 240.

10. Kudrow, L. (1980). In: Cluster headache: mechanisms and management.
    pp. 21-39. (Oxford: University Press).

11. Nappi, G. and Savoldi, F. In: Le Cefalee: sistema diagnostico e
    classificazione. pp. 82-89. (Milano: Workshop Italiana).

12. Manzoni, G.C., Terzano, M.G., Bono, G. Micieli, G., Martucci, N.
    and Nappi, G. (1982). Clinical findings and natural history of 180

patients with cluster headache. Cephalalgia, 3, 21-30.

13. Kudrow, L. (1980). In: Cluster headache: mechanisms and management. pp. 71-99. (Oxford: University Press).

14. Mandell, A.J. and Knapp, S. (1979). Asymmetry and mood, emergent properties of serotonin regulation. Arch. Gen. Psychiatry, 36, 909-16.

15. Russel, D. and von der Lippe, A. (1982). Cluster Headache: heart rate and blood pressure changes during spontaneous attacks. Cephalalgia, 2, 61-70.

16. Sjaastad, O. and Saunte, C. (1982). Sweating in cluster headache: patterns and possible underlying mechanisms. In: Clifford Rose (ed.). Advances in migraine research and therapy. pp. 67-78. (New York: Raven Press).

17. Sandrini, G., Micieli, G., Martignoni, E., Savoldi, F. and Nappi, G. (1983). Unilateral impairment of pupillary responsiveness to noxious stimulation of sural nerve in episodic cluster headache. 1st Internat. Headache Congress, Munich, Sept. 14-16, 1983. (Abstract book, p. 102).

18. Nappi, G., Facchinetti, F., Bono, G., Petraglia, F., Micieli, G., Cicoli, C. and Genazzani, A.R. (1983). Lack of B-endorphin circadian rhythm in cluster headache: a model for chronopathology. Ibidem (p. 31-2).

19. Ekbom, K. (1981). Lithium for cluster headache: review of the literature and preliminary results of long term treatment. Headache, 21, 132-9.

20. Katz, R.J. and Carrol, B.J. (1977). Effects of chronic lithium and rubidium administration upon experimentally induced conflict behavior. Progr. Neuro-Psychopharmacol., 1, 285-91.

21. Meltzer, H.L., Taylor, R.M., Platman, S.R. and Fieve, R.R. (1969). Rubidium: a potential modifier of affect and behavior. Nature, 223, 321.

22. Gottesfeld, Z., Samuel, D. and Ycekson, Y. (1973). Glutamate and

GABA levels and glutamate decarboxylase activity in brain regions of rats after prolonged treatment with alkali cations. <u>Experientia</u>, <u>29</u>, 68.

23.Carolei, A., Sonsini, V., Casacchia, M., Agnoli, A. and Fazio, C. (1975). Azione farmacologica del cloruro di rubidio. Effetto anti-depressivo: confronto con l'imipramina. <u>La Clin. Terap.</u>, <u>75</u>, 469-73.

24. Chouinard, G. and Annable, L. (1977). Effects of rubidium in schizophrenia. <u>Commun. Psycho-pharmacol.</u>, <u>1</u>, 373-76.

25
Lithium therapy in cluster headache. Effect on iris neuromuscular junction

M. FANCIULLACCI, U. PIETRINI, M. BOCCUNI and F. SICUTERI

The effectiveness of lithium treatment in chronic cluster headache(CH) is now well documented (1-4). It remains to established however,if the drug is effective in episodic CH (5,6). This point is of particular importance considering that approximately 90% of patients are of episodic type. Additionally, if the effect of lithium therapy supports a primary central pathogenesis of CH (7), the exact therapeutic mechanism of lithium therefore is obscure.
This chapter summarizes our clinical experiences with lithium therapy and its influence on the iris neuromuscular junction.

LITHIUM THERAPY

Analysis of our clinical experiences indicates various considerations. The effectiveness of lithium in CH has been evaluated in 76 patients(20 with the chronic form and 56 with the episodic form).These patients presented with the typical clinical features of CH syndrome. All showed a positive response to the diagnostic pupillary tyramine test (8,9). Patients were treated with lithium carbonate doses ranging from 600-1200 mg/die for 6 to 12 months, which maintained the serum lithium levels between 0.4 and 0.9 mEq/l.In 14 patients with chronic CH lithium provoked an absolute or partial improvement of the syndrome.The other 6 patients without the benefit of lithium carbonate were treated with slow release lithium sulphate (600-1200 mg/die)resulting in a partial benefit for 4. Prophylactic treatment with lithium carbonate was performed in seasonal well-timed CH patients in whom the length and frequency of previous period were excellent parameters for evaluating the effectiveness of the drug. Preventive effectiveness was observed in the majority of these patients as lithium was capable of preventig the recurrence of clusters or attenuating the frequency and intensity of attacks. In episodic CH

with bizarre and bad timed active phases and with prologed remissions therapeutic efficacy of litnium in preventing the cluster period cannot be discriminated from spontaneous remissions. In these cases prophyla-xis appears not to be opportune,however, beginning treatment at the first attack of the cluster may result in a partial improvement.
Lithium therapy is well tolerated also in long term use and the medica-tion rarely must be discontinuated.

EFFECT OF LITHIUM ON IRIS NEUROMUSCULAR JUNCTION

Eleven CH patients were followed for 6 months with lithium carbonate treatment (900 mg/die).
Pupils were statistically isocoric for the entire period of observation

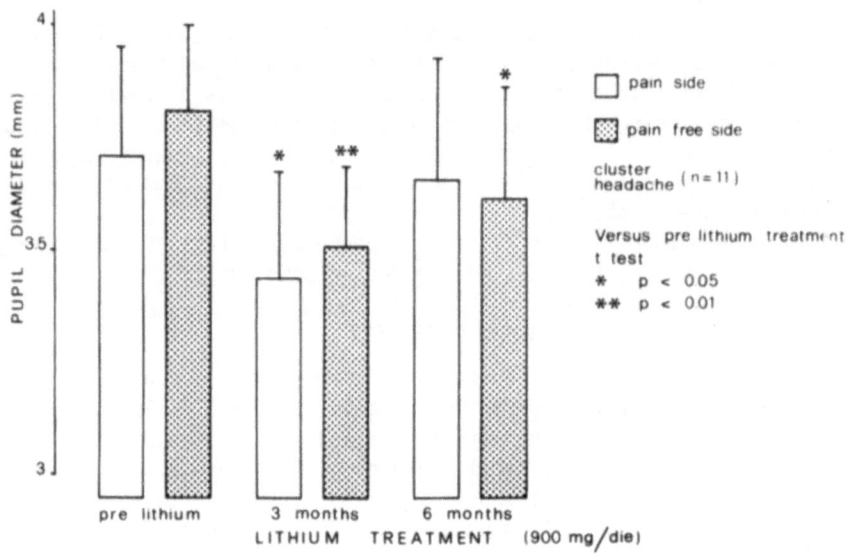

Fig 1. Pupil size during lithium therapy in CH.In brackets number of patients studied. Means ± SEM

After 3 months of treatment a significant decrease of pupil size was ob̲ served in both eyes. After 6 months however,the pupil of the asymptoma-tic side remained decreased (Fig 1).
In CH patients one eye drop of 2% tyramine,a norepinephrine (NE) relea-ser, instilled into both eyes, induced an anisocoric mydriasis. This is

due to a less marked response on the symptomatic side. In 6 patients
suffering from chronic CH the tyramine-induced anisocoria disappeared
after 4 months of lithium treatment, since mydriatic response to tyramine on the asymptomatic side was reduced,and that of the pain side was
increased (Fig 2). One patient tested at 2 months intervals showed at

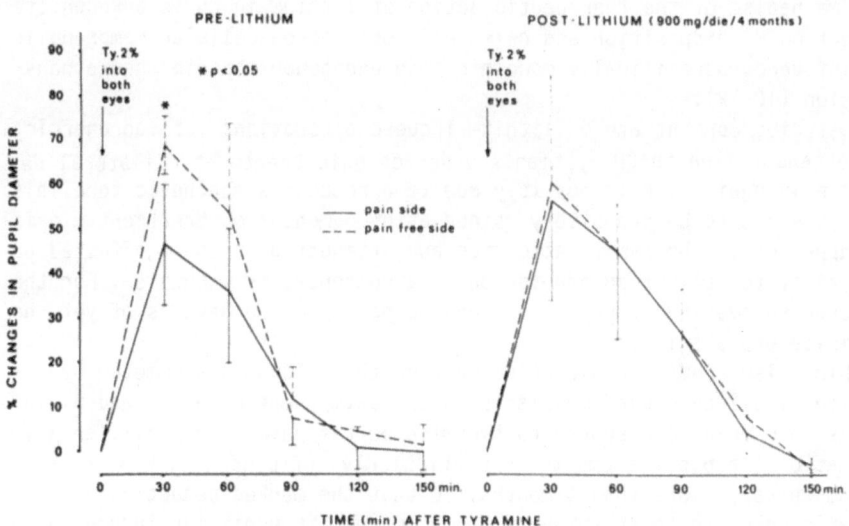

Fig 2. Tyramine-induced mydriasis before and after lithium
treatment. Lithium corrects tyramine-induced anisocoria.
Means ± SEM of 6 chronic CH patients; p between the two
pupils.

both 6 and 8 months an inverted anisocoria due to a response that was
markedly reduced on the pain-free side.Improvement of the headache corresponded to the restoration of a well balanced response to tyramine.

DISCUSSION

It has been our experience, as well as that of other authors, to observe a maximal therapeutic effectiveness of lithium in chronic CH. In some cases however, lithium treatment failed to improve the syndrome. Benefit was also obtained with slow release tablets supporting the idea

that occasionally the lack of effectiveness of lithium carbonate may partially be due to the decrease of its blood concentrations between ad ministrations.

Lithium-induced improvement in episodic CH is difficult to distinguish from spontaneous remissions,particularly if clusters occur irregularly. However, with our menagement technique, i.e. starting treatment at the first attack of cluster, evaluation of therapeutic action is possible. With this procedure the benefit is only partial but not less than that observed with other drugs.

The mechanism of the therapeutic action of lithium in CH is unknown.Its effect on NE disposition and release as well as on cellular membrane is to influence aspecifically monoamine and endogenous opioid neurotransmission (10-12).

Our studies concentrate on lithium-induced alterations of adrenergic nurotransmission in CH patients under chronic treatment. Bilateral decrease in pupil size is possibly due to a reduced sympatnetic tone.This effect seems to be transitory, since after 6 months of treatment miosis disappeared on the symptomatic side and attenuated on the unaffected pu pil,as if to reflect an adaptation of a compensatory mechanism. For the quicker recovering of pupil size on the pain side we have as of yet no definite explanation.

Lithium also seems capable of correcting the autonomic asymmetry by reducing tyramine-induced mydriasis on the asymptomatic pupil and by increasing mydriatic response to tyramine on the pain-side pupil.The asym ptomatic side pupil seems to be particularly influenced by prolonged li thium therapy (more than 4 months) so that the marked reduction of mydriatic response to tyramine of the asymptomatic pupil may induce an in verted asymmetry.

Since the well balanced autonomic activity corresponds to the clinical improvement of CH syndrome, it is postulated that lithium corrects the neuronal asymmetries which provoke a lateralization of both autonomic dysfunction and pain.

High concentrations of the drug found in the hypothalamus and its influ ence on both sleep patterns and circadian rhythms (13,14), which are al tered in CH (15,16), support the concept that lithium may act on latera lized pain as well as on sympathergic asymmetry, modifiyng neuronal transmission in central nervous system. Further evidence is offered by lithium's capability of reducing bilateral asymmetry in serotonin content at mesostriatal and mesolimbic levels (17). Recent data demonstrate a physiological bilateral asymmetry of aminergic and peptidergic activity at cortical and subcortical levels (18-21). An amplification of physiological asymmetry may cause diseases as has been postulated particularly in manic depressive syndrome with bipolar affective disorders (17) and in cluster headache both of which are improved by lithium therapy.

Aknowledgements. This work was supported by a grant from CNR (Rome)

Finalized Project on Preventative Medicine, group Pain Control.

REFERENCES

1. Ekbom K. (1974) Lithium vid kronska symptom av cluster headache.Opus Med. 19:148-156.

2. Kudrow L. (1977) Lithium prophylaxis for chronic cluster headache. Headache 17:15-18.

3. Mathew N.T. (1978) Clinical subtypes of cluster headache and response to lithium therapy. Headache 18:26-30.

4. Klimek A. , Szule-Kuberska T. and Kawiorski S. (1979) Lithium therapy in cluster headache. Eur.Neurol. 18:267-268.

5. Ekbom K. (1981) Lithium for cluster headache: review of the litterature and preliminary results of long-term treatment. Headache 21:132 -139.

6. Manzoni G.C., Bono G., Lanfranchi M., Micieli G., Terzano M.G. and Nappi G. (1983) Lithium carbonate in cluster headache: assessment of its short- and long-term therapeutic efficacy. Cephalalgia 3: 109-114.

7. Sjaastad O. (1978) pathogenesis of the cluster headache syndrome.Res Clin. Stud. Headache 6:53-64.

8. Fanciullacci M., Boccuni M., Pietrini U. and Cangi F. (1982) Pupilla ry tyramine test: its disgnostic relevance in cluster headache. Pan. Med 24:81-83.

9. Fanciullacci M., Pietrini U., Gatto G., Boccuni M. and Sicuteri F. (1982) Latent dysautonomic pupillary lateralization in cluster headache.A pupillometric study. Cephalalgia 2:135-144.

10.Katz R.I.,Kopin I.J. (1969) Release of norepinephrine-^{3}H and serotonin-^{3}H evoked from brain slices by electric field stimulation. Calcium dependence and the effct of lithium, ouabain, and tetrodoxin. Biochem. Pharmacol 18:1935-1939.

11.Beaty O., Colis M.G., Shepherd J.T. (1981) Action of lithium on adre nergic nerve ending. J.Pharmacol.Exp.Ther. 218:309-317.

12.Gillin J.C., Hong S,Yang H.Y.T., Costa E. (1978) Enkephalin content in brain regions of rats treated with lithium. Proc. Natl.Acad. Sci. USA 75:2991-2993.

13.Chernik D.A., Cochran C,Mendels J. (1974) Effects of lithium carbona te on sleep. J.Psychitr.Res 10:133-146.

14.Kripke D.,Wyborney 'V.G. (1980) Lithium slows rat circadian rhythms. Life Sci. 26:1319-1321.

15. Nappi G., Ferrari E., Polleri A.,Savoldi F.,Vailati A. (1981) Chro-
    nobiological study in cluster headache. Chronobiologia 2: 140.

16. Polleri A., Nappi G., Murialdo G., Bono G., Martignoni E. Savoldi
    F. (1982) Changes in 24-h prolactin pattern in cluster headache.Ce-
    phalalgia 2:1-7.

17. Mandel A.J. and Knapp S. (1979) Asymmetry and mood;emergent proper-
    ties of serotonin regulation. Arch.Gen.Psychiatry 20:909-916.

18. Glick S.D.,Jerussi T.P. and Fleicher L.N. (1976) Turning in circles
    : the neuropharmacology of rotation. Life sci 18:889-896.

19. Oke A., Keller R., Hefford J. and Adams R.N. (1978) Lateralization
    in norepinephrine in human thalamus. Science 200:1411-1413.

20. Amaducci L.,Sorbi S., Albanese A. and Gainotti G. (1981) Choline a-
    cetyltransferase (ChAT) activity differs in right and left human
    temporal lobes. Neurology 31: 799-805.

21. Chasov E.I., Bakalkin G.Y., Yarigin K.N., Trushina E.D., Titov M.I.
    and Smirnov V.N. (1981) Enkephalins induce asymmetrical effects on
    in the rat. Experientia 37:887-889.

26
Changes in tubular enzymes during acute lithium treatment

A. LENZI, M. TUONI, E. RAMPELLO, R. PALLA, P. FORNARO AND G. F. PLACIDI

In current psychiatric practice Lithium represents an indispensable therapeutic tool, as it has been shown to be the most active drug for the prophylaxis of recurrent affective bipolar disorders. Together with an increasing use of Lithium, there has been a higher frequency (1) of polyuria and polydipsia, indicating that nephrotoxicity may be involved.

The exact mechanism of the genesis of Lithium-induced natruresis and polyuria has not yet been precisely defined. It has been hypothesized that there is a competitive inhibition with sodium transport in the distal tubule, although this has not been demonstrated in man, or, perhaps, an interaction of Lithium with one or more of the systemic homeostatic mechanisms that control the reabsorption of renal sodium. Inhibition of renal sodium appears to be ADH-mediated, although no demonstration of such inhibition has been given in man. Finally, there appears to be an inhibition of the system of renin-angiotensin-aldosterone. During chronic Lithium therapy the activity of plasma renin and aldosterone levels appears to show normal limits; controversy exists as to the nature of these parameters during states of Lithium toxicity (4).

Although it has been noted for over 20 years that alteration of kidney function may be associated with Lithium therapy, it has only recently been hypothesized that permanent renal damage (4) (5) may result. A number of investigators have noted that a Lithium-induced fall in renal concentration capacity became less severe after the interruption of therapy, but this capacity seems to persist at rather lower levels than in normals (2) (3) (4) (5).

Two mechanisms for this fall in renal concentrating capacity have been hypothesized. The first is dose-related, and is apparently mediated by the suppression of ADH activity on renal tubules. The second is daily dose-independent and is correlated with the total dose received during the entire course of treatment, the duration of treatment, and the maximum levels administered, and could lead to apparently permanent structural changes within the nephron (5) (6).

The histological sections of renal needle-biopsy material taken from patients who had normal renal function before Lithium treatment and who had then been treated for 2 years with Lithium showed (2) (3) (4) that almost 25% of the patients show signs of a chronic interstitial nephropathy associated with a fall in renal concentrating capacity (7). These sections have shown cortical and medullary focal interstitial fibrositis with marked atrophy of the nephron and moderate infiltration of mononuclear cells. These findings, however, remain inconclusive, as there was no homogeneous control group and no definitively demonstrated pathological mechanisms capable to accounting for these changes.

Since further evaluation of the nephrotoxic action of Lithium was needed to inquire deeper into the possible pathogenetic mechanism, it seemed that besides the usual renal laboratory examinations, analyses should be carried out on enzymes such as gamma-GT, muramidase and alfa-glucosidase, which are early sensitive and reliable indicators of renal damage (8) (9) (10).

We therefore decided to evaluate changes in various renal enzymes in patients in whom Lithium therapy was indicated as a suitable form of treatment. A 10 cc blood sample and a 24-hours urine sample were collected from each of 15 female inpatients. None of these patients had had previous Lithium therapy, but all were currently on various antidepressant or neureleptic treatments. These samples were obtained prior to and immediately after a 30-day Lithium trial. The data obtained by us from the standard renal laboratory examinations before and after Lithium treatment seemed to conform to those reported by other authors. We found a significant increase in diuresis, of BUN clearance and natruresis (Table 1).

These samples were studied for changes in certain renal tubular enzymes (11): alfa-glucosidase (13), muramidase (12) and renal gamma-GT; a rise in their concentration reflects renal tubular damage. All the enzymes studied demonstrated a rise in urinary concentration in their post-treatment levels when compared to their baseline values.

Alfa-glucosidase initially presented values at the upper limits of the normal range and at post-treatment analysis showed levels in the frankly pathologic range.

LABORATORY FINDINGS BEFORE (I) AND AFTER THIRTY DAYS (II) LITHIUM SALTS TREATMENT

LAB.	I		II		p
	MEAN	S.D.	MEAN	S.D.	
DIURESIS (ml)	1625	532	1794	686	.05
S. CREATININE (mg%)	0.84	0.145	0.84	0.125	--
Cr. Cl. (ml/min)	105.56	34	105.8	32	--
B.U.N. (mg%)	32.27	8.71	28	9.14	--
B.U.N. Cl. (ml/min)	35.57	15.4	53.18	20.6	.05
URIC AC. - EMIA (mg%)	4.09	1.31	4.16	0.99	--
URIC AC. - URIA (mg/24h)	558.89	131.17	573.85	231.4	--
Na - EMIA (meq/l)	138.6	2.847	140.13	2.276	--
Na - URIA (meq/24h)	160.78	35.168	166.72	73	.05
K - EMIA (meq/l)	3.97	0.37	4.25	0.34	--
K - URIA (meq/24h)	84.73	11.1	71.16	36.24	--
Ca - EMIA (meq/l)	4.65	0.43	4.68	0.38	--
Ca - URIA (meq/24h)	7.47	3.93	9.01	4.35	--
P - EMIA (meq/l)	1.74	0.29	1.75	0.39	--
P - URIA (meq/24h)	18.54	10.54	18.77	9.64	--
ph	7.385	0.025	7.4	0.029	--
HCO3	23.28	1.663	23.7	1.43	--
PCO2	39.54	2.026	38.81	2.19	--

The same relationship was noted for renal muramidase (Table 2).

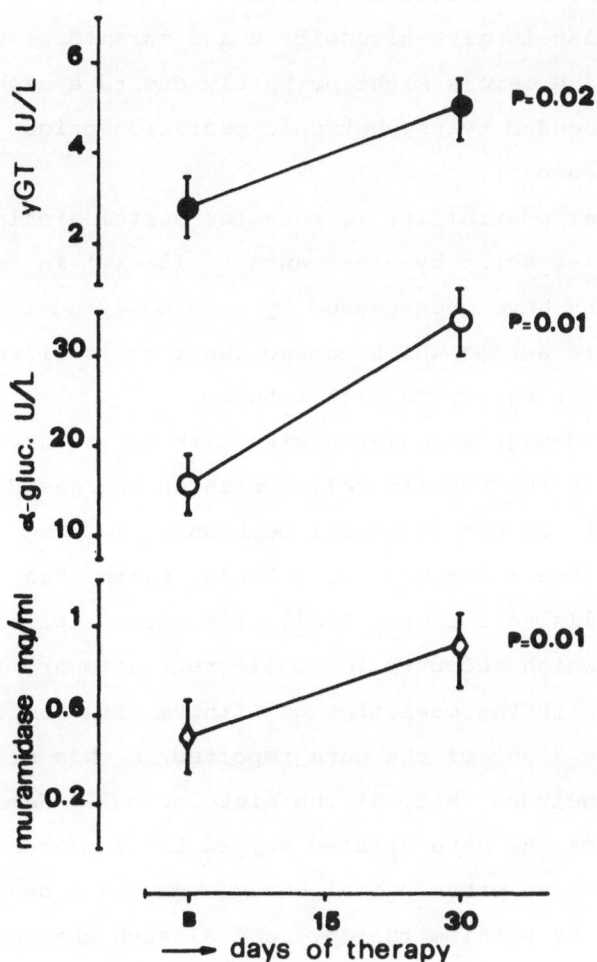

The levels recorded for the gamma-GT enzyme went from
midrange normal to upper limits of normal. The results of
this study seem to imply damaging effects to the kidney, at
least at the intracellular level.

The rise in alfa-glucosidase and muramidase values
above basline levels might be partly due to a nephrotoxic
effect proceeded by psychotropic mediation prior to
Lithium treatment.

Another possibility is that the histological
abnormalities noted by other authors (5) (7) in renal
biopsies may have been caused by previously administered
psychotropic agents which caused their toxic effect either
alone or in conjunction with Lithium.

Renal damage associated with Lithium therapy appears
primarily in the tubular cells, with an increased
permeability of the lysosomal membranes, leading to the
release of their enzymes and cellular death. The renal
tubular cells have a practically limitless replication
capacity, which accounts for their return toward functional
normality with the cessation of Lithium treatment.

In the light of the data reported in this study, it
must be concluded that: 1) the histologically demonstrated
renal damage may have existed before Lithium treatment
began, 2) these pathological changes may have been
aggravated by Lithium therapy, and 3) such changes might
be the result of pre-treatment with other psychotropic
compounds.

References

1) SCHOU M. (1958)   : Lithium studies.
Acta Pharmacol. Toxicol. 15: 85-124.

2) SINGER I. (1981)   : Lithium and kidney.
Kidney International 19: 374-387.

3) DE PAULO R., CORREA E.I., SAPIR D.G. (1981) : Renal toxicity of lithium and its implications.
John Hopkins Medical Journal 149: 15-21.

4) ALEXANDER F., MARTIN J. (1980) : Lithium and the nephrotic syndrome.
Lab. Invest. 42: 97.

5) BUCHT G., WAHLIN A. (1980): Renal concentrating capacity in long-term lithium treatment and after with drawal of lithium.
Acta Med. Scand. 207: 309-314.

6) THOMSEN K. (1976)   : Renal elimination of lithium in rats with lithium intoxication.
J. Pharm. Ther. 199: 483-489.

7) VESTERGAARD P., AMDISEN A., HANSEN H.E., SCHOU M. (1979)   : Lithium treatment and kidney function.

Acta Psychiat. Scand. 60: 504-520.

8) GARVEY M.J., VICENTE B., TUASON M., CHARLES H., BLOMQUIST, SUTAEG H. (1982) : Evaluation of nephrotoxicity in affective disorders using renal enzymes.
Br. J. Psychiatry Oct.

9) KINCAID SMITH P., BURROWS G.D., DAVIES B., HOLWILL B., WALTER M., WALKER R. (1979) : Renal biopsy findings in lithium and pre-lithium patients.
Lancet 2: 700-701.

10) PRICE R.G. (1982) : Urinary enzymes, nephrotoxicity and renal disease.
Toxicoloty 23: 99-134.

11) BONINI P.A. (1970) : Human urinary alfa-glucosidase as an index of kidney tubular damage.
Clin. Chim. Acta 27: 15-29.

12) SZASZ G. (1974) : Gamma-glutamyl-transpeptidase.
In: Begmeyer H.V. Ed. Methods of enzymatic analysis.
New York Academic Press 715-722.

13) PROCKOP D.J. (1964) : A study of urinary and serum lysozyme in patients with renal disease.
N.England J.Med 270: 269-274

27
Prophylactic efficacy of carbamazepine in lithium-resistant affective disorders

M. DEL ZOMPO, C. BURRAI, M. P. PICCARDI, A. MARELLI AND G. U. CORSINI

Several clinical studies have confirmed the efficacy of lithium salts in mania and in the prevention of recurrent attacks of manic-depressive illness (1,2,3,4). However, not all patients benefit from this therapy. Furthermore, due to toxic side-effects, the periodic measurement of lithium serum levels during treatment is necessary. Thus, the possibility of conceiving alternative drugs with antimanic and prophylactic effects similar to those of lithium is desirable.

Carbamazepine (Tegretol), an iminodibenzyl derivative which is considered the treatment of choice for trigeminal neuralgia (5,6) and has also been reported to be effective in other pain syndromes (6,7,8), might be taken into consideration for this hypothesis.

This drug is a well-known anticonvulsant with remarkable effectiveness in seizure disorders involving temporal lobe and limbic area in animals and man (9, 10,11). The clinical evidence of psychotropic effects of carbamazepine (CBZ) in mood and behavioural disorders, whether associated (9,12) or not (13,14,15) with complex partial seizures, is noteworthy. Therefore, the demonstrated therapeutic efficacy of CBZ in patients with seizure-related mood disorders suggested the clinical usefulness of this drug in patients with non-seizure mood disorders.

Recently, many investigators have observed that CBZ may be effective in manic-depressive patients (16,17,18,19). We report here a one year study with 10 manic-depressive patients who have to date completed the clinical trial. These preliminary data confirm the usefulness of carbamazepine on therapy and on prophylaxis of affective illness.

MATERIALS AND METHODS.

We studied 10 patients (8 males and 2 females) aged between 24 - 67 years. Diagnoses were formed according to Diagnostic Statistical Manual III (DSM III) as follows: Major Depression, recurrent (1 patient); Bipolar Manic Disorder (6 patients); Manic episode (1 patient); Bipolar Disorder, Depressive (1 patient); Bipolar Disorder, Mixed (1 patient). Patients were admitted to the study if they had past history of lithium or neuroleptic non-response or serious side effects related to lithium treatment. All patients underwent neurological examinations and tests in order to rule out the possibility of seizure disorders.

All these patients were treated with carbamazepine at an initial dosage of 200 mg per day, which was however gradually increased every 5 days until a maximum daily dosage of 1200 - 1600 mg was achieved or a clinical effect was obtained. The CBZ blood levels were constantly monitored and the levels were generally maintained within the range of 8 - 12 µg/ml. Moreover, the presence of both clinical and haematological side effects was evaluated. Patients were evaluated approximately every two months or, in any case, when relapse occurred, with the BPRS Psychiatric Rating Scale (20) for 1 year. In all patients, the prophylactic trial progressed in an open design and the efficacy of carbamazepine was evaluated by the incidence of affective episodes during the trial compared to the previous year. We here describe briefly the clinical history of each patient:

1) P.I., a 56 year old female. She had a 7 year history of recurring depressive episodes with a marked state of anxiety and psychomotor agitation. These episodes were manifested on an average of 2 per year. The patient was treated with lithium + tricyclics for 4 years, but with no clinical improvement. She has been taking CBZ (600 mg per day) for one year and during this period has not presented any further depressive episodes.

2) P.P., a 67 year old male. Over the last 10 years, he had presented recurrent manic episodes on an average of 3 per year. The patient had been treated previously with neuroleptics with no beneficial effect. He has been under CBZ therapy (600 mg per day) + haloperidol for 14 months. Since this therapy was started, the patient has not presented manic or depressive episodes. The presence of side effects (occasional dizziness) has been described.

3) S.S., a 45 year old male. He has presented one manic episode in the last year which was unaffected by neuroleptic treatment. For one year he has been under therapy with CBZ (600 mg per day) and has since been euthymic with no side effects.

4) T.I., a 50 year old male. He had a 10 year history of alternating recurrent manic and depressive episodes with an average frequency of 2 per year. In the last 3 years he had been under therapy with lithium + neuroleptics with poor therapeutic results. Since he has been under CBZ (600 mg per day) and haloperidol, he has only presented one brief depressive episode and no side effects.

5) F.G., a 30 year old male. For more than 10 years he had presented alternating depressive and manic episodes on an average of 1.5 per year. Treatment with lithium + neuroleptics did not result in an improvement of the psychiatric status. He has been taking CBZ (600 mg per day) alone for the last 15 months. One month after the beginning of this therapy, the patient presented a mild depressive episode which was rapidly resolved without additional therapy. Since then, he has been euthymic and has not been subjected to any side effects.

6) A.V., a 32 year old female with a 10 year history of alternating manic and depressive episodes, with an average frequency of 3 per year. Six years of therapy with lithium + neuroleptics did not offer any significant improvement. She has been in therapy for one year with CBZ (600 mg per day). The patient has presented no further episodes and the only side effect was nausea which however disappeared as therapy progressed.

7) C.V., a 58 year old male. This patient had a 10 year history of numerous serious depressive and manic episodes with an average frequency of 2 per year.

He had been treated with lithium salts for 4 years but with no beneficial effect. Over the last year the patient had been taking CBZ (1200 mg per day). After starting this therapy, he has not presented any new episodes. The therapy caused the onset of side effects such as nausea and dyspepsia.

8) M.A., a 24 year old male. He had suffered from numerous manic episodes on an average of 2.5 per year. Four years of lithium treatment + neuroleptics had not improved the clinical picture. For 14 months he has been under treatment with CBZ (800 mg per day) + neuroleptics. During this period he has presented 2 brief manic episodes and no side effects.

9) O.G., a 38 year old male. Over the last 8 years, the patient had presented numerous rapid cycles of manic and depressive episodes, with an average frequency of 3 per year. These episodes were accompanied by delusions and marked loss of association and illogical thinking. Treatment with lithium salts and neuroleptics did not modify the symptomatology. The patient has been taking CBZ (1200 mg per day) + neuroleptics for 13 months. During this period he has presented 2 manic episodes and 1 depressive one, having the same features as the previous ones. As side effect, drowsiness was observed which disappeared as therapy continued.

10) D.P., a 36 year old male. He had a 6 year history of periodic manic episodes on an average of 2 per year. Previously treated with lithium + neuroleptics with no beneficial clinical result; he is now under therapy with CBZ (600 mg per day) + haloperidol. After 3 months of treatment, he presented a brief manic episode and has since been euthymic.

Diagnoses and previous treatment of all patients admitted to the trial are summarized in Table 1.

TABLE 1

CASE	AGE	SEX	DIAGNOSIS (DSM III)	PREVIOUS TREATMENT
1	56	F	MAJOR DEPRESSION	LITHIUM + TRICYCLICS
2	67	M	BIPOLAR DISORDER MANIC	NEUROLEPTICS
3	45	M	BIPOLAR DISORDER MANIC	NEUROLEPTICS
4	50	M	BIPOLAR DISORDER MANIC	LITHIUM + NEUROLEPTICS
5	30	M	BIPOLAR DISORDER MANIC	LITHIUM + NEUROLEPTICS
6	32	F	BIPOLAR DISORDER MANIC	LITHIUM + NEUROLEPTICS
7	58	M	BIPOLAR DISORDER DEPRESSED	LITHIUM
8	24	M	BIPOLAR DISORDER MANIC	LITHIUM + NEUROLEPTICS
9	38	M	BIPOLAR DISORDER MIXED	LITHIUM + NEUROLEPTICS
10	36	M	BIPOLAR DISORDER MANIC	LITHIUM + NEUROLEPTICS

RESULTS AND DISCUSSION

As summarized in Table 2, 6 out of 10 patients showed a good prophylactic response to carbamazepine. In the year prior to CBZ treatment the patients had been affected by an average of 3.15 episodes of mania or depression. During CBZ prophylaxis they presented only 0.8 episodes per year of therapy (paired t = 6.06 p = < .001). When episodes did occur during carbamazepine treatment, they were generally less severe and shorter lasting than previous episodes. We should underline how patients treated with CBZ who also needed association with neuroleptics, never required such high doses of the drugs as in previous episodes.

TABLE 2.   Prophylactic efficacy of Carbamazepine in cyclical affective illness.

CASE	DURATION OF TREATM.	CBZ BLOOD LEVELS (ug/ml)	OTHER DRUGS	TOTAL EPISODES**		SIDE EFFECTS
				BEFORE	CBZ	
1	12	10.5	–	2.5	0	NONE
2	14	9.6	HALOPERIDOL	4	0	DIZZINESS
3	12	9.0	–	1	0	NONE
4	12.5	8.5	HALOPERIDOL	4	1	NONE
5	15	10.5	–	3	1	NONE
6	12	6.7	–	3.5	0	NAUSEA
7	11	12.3	–	4	0	NAUSEA
8	14.5	9.0	NEUROLEPTICS	3	2	–
9	13	8.5	NEUROLEPTICS	4	3	DROWSINESS
10	13	7.6	HALOPERIDOL	2.5	1	–
	12.9 + 1.26	9.22 + 1.6		3.15 +.97*	0.8 + 1.03*	

* Paired t = 6.06 p < 0.001   ** Before = episodes during the year prior CBZ
                                     CBZ = episodes/year during CBZ treatment

The plasma levels of CBZ in these patients were within the range considered therapeutic for the epileptic patients, between 6.7 and 12.35 μg/ml with a mean value of 9.22 + 1.6 μg/ml. In spite of the high levels of CBZ reached, patients 8 and 9 have not shown any appreciable improvement. Side effects such as nausea, dyspepsia, dizziness, drowsiness and exanthema which were observed during carbamazepine treatment did not require interruption of therapy. There was no evidence of blood test abnormalities.

These data obtained in a small number of patients, in agreement with those reported in literature, confirm the therapeutic efficacy of carbamazepine in affective disorders. The present study concerned only lithium and neuroleptic non-responders, although some authors have reported that CBZ may benefit previous lithium responders also (18,19). However, we suggest that the clinical usefulness of carbamazepine today is most important in lithium non-responders and in this way, as in other studies (21), we obtained promising results.

A correlation between blood levels of carbamazepine and clinical efficacy of the drug was not found. A possible explanation could be that the carbamazepine metabolite considered to be active in epilepsy is the 10-11 epposside. The availability of dosage methods for this metabolite will further clear its importance in the explanation of the clinical efficacy of CBZ in affective disorders. These data might suggest that measurement of serum levels of CBZ in affective disorders could be of limited value.

In conclusion, our study underlined the fact that carbamazepine may be used with fewer side effects than lithium and requires less frequent clinical pharmacological controls.

Some authors suggested that carbamazepine's clinical efficacy in affective disorders could be related to its action on limbic structures (22). Moreover, some studies suggested that CBZ inhibits noradrenaline sensitive adenylate cyclase in brain (23) as does lithium (24) and, recently, some authors demonstrated a specific and potent interaction of CBZ with brain adenosine receptors (25). We retain that the discovery of the mechanism of action of receptor sites of CBZ will allow us to obtain answers to old and new questions on the biochemical aethiology of some mental disorders.

REFERENCES

1) Cade J.F. Lithium salts in the treatment of psychotic excitement. Med.J.Aust. 36, 349-352, 1949.
2) Johnson G., Gershon S., Burdock E., Floyd A., Hekimian L.: Comparative effects of lithium and chlorpromazine in the treatment of acute manic states". Br.J. Psychiatry 119, 267-276, 1971.
3) Prien R.F., Caffey E.M.Jr., Klett C.J.: Comparison of lithium carbonate and chlorpromazine in the treatment of mania. Arch.Gen.Psychiatry 26, 146-153, 1972.
4) Prien R.F., Caffey E.M.Jr., Klett C.J. : Relationship between serum lithium level and clinical response in acute manic treated with lithium. Br.J.Psychiatry, 120, 409-414, 1972.
5) Blom S.: Trigeminal neuralgia: its treatment with a new anticonvulsant drug G32883. Lancet I, 839-840, 1962.
6) Killian J.M. and Fromm G.H.: Carbamazepine (Tegretol) in the treatment of neuralgia: use and side effects. Arch.Neurol. 19, 129-136, 1968.
7) Davis E.H.: Clinical trials of Tegretol R in trigeminal neuralgia. Headache 9, 77-82, 1969.
8) Yang C.P. and Nagaswami S.: Cardiac syncope secondary to glossopharyngeal neuralgia effectively treated with carbamazepine. J.Clin.Psychiatry 39, 776-778, 1978.
9) Dalby M.A.: Antiepileptic and psychotropic effects of carbamazepine (Tegretol) in the treatment of psychomotor epilepsy. Epilepsia 12, 325-334, 1971.
10) Penry J.K. and Daly D.D.: Complex Partial Seizures: Adv.in Neurology, Vol.II, Raven Press, New York, 1975.
11) Rodin E.A., Rim C.S., Rennick P.M.: The effects of carbamazepine on patients with psychomotor epilepsy: results of a double blind study. Epilepsia 15, 547-561, 1974.

12) Dalby M.A.: Behavioural effects of carbamazepine. In: Penry J.K. and Daly D.D. (Eds.), Complex Partial Seizures, Adv.Neurology Vol.II, Raven Press, New York, 1975.

13) Kuhn R.: The psychotropic effect of carbamazepine in non-epileptic adults with particular reference to the drug's possible mechanism of action. In: Epileptic Seizures - Behaviour - Pain. Ed: W.Birkmayer, Hans Huber Publ., pp.32-48, 1975.

14) Kuhn-Gebhart V.: Behavioural disorders in non epileptic children and their treatment with carbamazepine. In: Epileptic Seizures - Behaviour - Pain. Ed: W.Birkmayer, Hans Huber Publ. pp.246-267, 1975.

15) Puente R.M.: The use of carbamazepine in the treatment of behavioural disorders in children. In: Eplieptic Seizures - Behaviour - Pain, Ed: W.Birkmayer, Hans Huber Publ. pp. 243-247, 1975.

16) Okuma T., Inanaga K., Otsuki S., Sarai K., Takahashi R., Hazama H., Mori A., Watanaba M.: Comparison of antimanic efficacy of carbamazepine and chlorpromazine: a double-blind controlled study. Psychopharmacology 66, 211-217, 1979.

17) Okuma T., Inanaga K., Otsuki S., Sarai A., Takahashi R., Hazama H., Mori A., Watanaba M.: A preliminary double-blind study on the efficacy of carbamazepine in the prophylaxis of manic-depressive illness. Psychopharmacology 73, 95-96, 1981.

18) Ballenger J.C., Post R.M.: Therapeutic effects of carbamazepine in affective illness. A preliminary report. Communications in Psychopharmacology 2, 159-175, 1978.

19) Ballenger J.C., Post R.M.: Carbamazepine in manic depressive illness: a new treatment. Am.J.Psychiatry 137, 782-790, 1980.

20) Overall J.E., Gorham D.R.: The brief psychiatric rating scale. Psychiatr. Rep 10, 799-812, 1962.

21) Klein E., Bental E., Lerer B., Belmaker R.H.: Combination of carbamazepine and haloperidol versus placebo and haloperidol in excited psychoses: a controlled study. Arch.Gen.Psych. In Press.

22) Post R.M.: Carbamazepine's acute and prophylactic effects in mania and depressive illness: An update. Intern.Drug Ther.Newsletter 17, 5-9, 1982.

23) Levine E., Bleck V.: Cyclic AMP-accumulation in cerebral cortical slices: effect of carbamazepine, phenobarbital and phenytoin. Epilepsia 18, 237-242, 1977.

24) Ebstein R., Belmaker R.H., Grunhaus L., Rimon R.: Lithium inhibition of adrenaline-stimulated adenylate cyclase in humans. Nature 259, 411-413, 1976

25) Marangos P.J., Post R.M., Patel J., Zander K., Parma A., Weiss S.: Specific and potent interactions of carbamazepine with brain adenosine receptors. Eur.J.Pharm.93, 175-182, 1983.

ACKNOWLEDGEMENTS

The authors wish to thank CIBA-GEIGY (Italy) for having provided the kits ne cessary for the dosage of the drug and for their invaluable technical assistance.

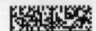